The

Happy

Hooker

ALSO BY XAVIERA HOLLANDER

The Happy Hooker

My Own Story

Xaviera Hollander

with **Robin Moore** and **Yvonne Dunleavy**

ReganBooks

An Imprint of HarperCollins*Publishers*

If you'd like to share your own comments or stories, E-mail can be sent directly to:

xaviera@xavierahollander.com

and check the Xaviera website for frequent updates:

www.xavierahollander.com

This book was originally published in 1972 by the Dell Publishing Group; a revised edition was first published in 1987 by Grafton Books and in 1995 by Diamond Books.

First ReganBooks paperback published 2002.

Designed by Sarah Maya Gubkin

Library of Congress Cataloging-in-Publication Data

Hollander, Xaviera.
 The happy hooker : my own story / Xaviera Hollander with Robin Moore and Yvonne Dunleavy.— 1st ReganBooks pbk.
  p. cm.
 Originally published: New York : Dell Pub. Co., ©1972. With new epilogue.
 ISBN 0-06-001416-4
  1. Hollander, Xaviera. 2. Prostitutes—United States—Biography
I. Moore, Robin, 1925– II. Dunleavy, Yvonne. III. Title.

HQ144.H64 2002
306.74'2'092—dc21   2002021265
[B]

02 03 04 05 06 ❖/RRD 10 9 8 7 6 5 4 3 2 1

Dedicated to
Larry and Takis

AUTHOR'S NOTE: The events in this book actually happened. The people actually exist. Only the names have been changed, and we genuinely regret any inadvertent similarity between these fictitious names and the names of real persons.

One

Rubber Souls

Almost from the moment we were herded into the crowded cattle pen of a prison cell in New York's infamous Tombs, the jail-toughened black hookers gave us nothing but misery.

"Hey, bigshit madambitch, bet you ain't got no black cunt turnin' tricks in your high-class fuckin' house!"

"Yeah, bet your midget-dick rich white johns can't buy no licorice from your candy store!"

"This queen bee of the hookers here, she afraid the black stuff gonna rub off all over her beeyootiful white sheets, ain't ya, honey?"

The hassling began bawdy, became ugly, then menacing.

"You there in the red-white-and-blue Saks fuckin' Fifth Avenue dress: Don't bend forward so far, otherwise ah'm gonna tear it off and eat you up!" Five minutes more and there could be a bloodbath, with us sure as hell the losers. There were seven of us, twenty of them, and common contempt of these street hookers for us, the expensive call girls, united them. In the hooker hierarchy, we were the aristocrats, they were the serfs, and jail, by God, was the great leveler.

I stood with my girls huddled tightly together against the cell bars, putting as much distance as possible between us and the black streetwalkers. Even if we wanted to sit down among the others, we had no chance. Those that had places on the few uncomfortable benches hung jealously on to them. If anyone got up for a drink of water or a pee, a fast ass would cancel the space. Some girls, exhausted from a night's sidewalk cruising, lay on the concrete floor, their heads in someone else's lap. They slept despite the anguished sounds of junkies in neighboring cells coughing, retching, and howling for relief. The stench of vomit, urine, and stale human body odor was suffocating.

The ranks oozed and abated like an oil slick as one group of girls, summoned by the big bull-dyke matron, was led to the courtroom and replaced with another. "Get over here, judge gonna see ya now."

Each new paddy wagon full of hookers fell in with the cat-calling. "Hey, muthafuckin' madam, can you tell us now why you don't have a little color in your high-class establishment?" a vicious-looking hooker in a neon-orange wig said menacingly.

Caution on my part gave way to exasperation, then anger. "Listen," I said, "I want you to know I do have black girls working for me. Several of them . . . I even have a black roommate. There she is over there."

I pointed to Aurora, a willowy light-skinned girl who was sitting apart from us. A prostitute since her teens, and the veteran of many arrests, the same experience that taught her how to grab a seat for herself also taught her to assume a low profile in this kind of a scene. Aurora sat in a corner, wearing a blond wig and dark glasses, her collar pulled high under her chin, trying to blend in with the walls. She squirmed as twenty pairs of eyes riveted on her.

The hookers stopped teasing their wigs and painting their nails with varnish that had mysteriously appeared despite all the handbags having been confiscated outside. "Sheeyit, man," a mean-looking coal-black girl finally rasped, "that mixed rat ain't black, she half-white."

"The scumbag dunno what the fuck she is," a girl with the face of a sepia madonna and the voice of a carnival barker said. Both she and her friend left their seats to walk toward Aurora for a better look and maybe take a swing at her. All of us were watching them. This had to be the moment of detonation.

Just then the cell gate cranked open, and the big black matron escorted in a fat white girl who was hobbling on crutches. The girl was all marked up with ulcers on her arms and legs and seemed to be dope-crazed. As the matron, in a kindly way, tried to ease her into one of the vacant seats, the girl yelled, "Take ya hands off me, ya big black dyke!" and hauled off, her crutch savagely ripping across the matron's head.

That was all we needed in this charged atmosphere, a racial explosion touched off by the handicapped whore. Girls started screaming and yelling; fists, arms, legs, and the crutches flew all over the place. My girls and I quickly moved for cover behind the urinal wall and waited to see what would happen next.

Three hefty matrons marched into the cell and efficiently subdued the hysterical white girl. What would happen next? Thank God we didn't have to hang around to find out. "Get over here, you girls behind the wall over there. Judge gonna see ya now." The cattle were led to the courtroom.

Inside the courtroom, full of journalists, quick-sketch artists, and curious onlookers, were my houseguests of the night before. The nice john from the Midwest I called Calvin was probably going to lose his job and marriage because his name and position had been blasted all over the New York papers. There was my sweet Greek lover, Takis, and beside him the couple whose only concession to convention was their last name. Otherwise they lived a life of free love and had been swinging with Takis and me in my house, for love, not money, only minutes before the cops arrived.

The judge listened with what seemed to me obvious hostility as the charges against us were read. One by one I paid the bail for my girls from the envelope of money I had stuffed into my panties before accompanying the cops to the station house. But the one person I wanted in the courtroom wasn't there: my boyfriend, Larry. I hadn't been able to contact him, and he had the key to the safe-deposit box where my main cash supply is kept. Now I was left without enough cash to pay the sky-high bail of $3,500 they put on "New York's most notorious madam"—as I heard myself described. So it was off to Riker's Island for me.

Riker's Island is the new women's prison, cleaner and more modern than the Tombs, but still the nesting place of the dregs of humanity. I was thrown into a big room full of junkies, pushers, ten-dollar harlots, the general hustlers of life, and victims of other people's crimes.

A scrawny white hooker who had been the victim of a "freak trick"—a customer who gets his kicks from brutally beating girls—was nursing her wounds. Three other hookers had been beaten by him on Eighth Avenue over the past two weeks, and this poor girl had bruises and cuts all over her, plus a broken arm and a lip which was cut to her nostril. Her eyes were swollen slits.

A sixteen-year-old Puerto Rican girl was crying for her three-week-old baby left unattended at home. "Mi marido try to kill me," she wailed in fractured English.

I tried to help the Spanish-speaking girls fill out their forms, but when I did, they would move away from me as though I had leprosy. So did the other prisoners. My expensive clothes and appearance made them suspicious and resentful.

They all stared, but nobody spoke to me except a cute little brown girl with freckles on a face like an acorn. "I have already been picked up eight times in two weeks," she said. "So now the judge decided to send me away for a month's rest."

She was agitated because her pimp did not know where she was. She wanted me to phone him when I got out.

When I got out? When would that be? It was 4:00 P.M. Friday, sixteen hours since my house was busted by three phony johns.

It is now daytime, so where is Larry with my bail money? Where is my lawyer? Why am I, a woman of class, happy in my profession and basically doing a necessary service, in this horrible place? I thought back on the bust, trying to understand where I had made my mistake.

Aurora could smell a cop a city block away. She didn't trust those three "clients" who had persistently phoned and insisted on coming over even though I tried to discourage them. We had been having a stag party earlier and now just a friendly social gathering. On their third call, around midnight, I finally allowed them to come up.

As soon as they came through the door, Aurora reacted like a gazelle downwind of a jackal. My instincts also signaled caution.

The swarthy man with the moustache sure looked like a john, and he was shaking in his shoes. The second one looked like a crook, and these days cops and crooks often look alike, so I couldn't be sure. But it was the third one, a tall man, who looked most like a cop.

"As a matter of routine," I said to them politely, "would you mind showing me some identification?" The one with the moustache shook some more, and he and Thugface looked toward the tall one, and he pulled a wallet from his pocket with only four of the dozen plastic compartments occupied. None of them contained credit cards. Cops can't afford credit cards. I didn't like it. I looked toward Aurora, who was staring down at the tall man's feet.

I followed her gaze. Rubber soles! The sure mark of a policeman. The cop followed our eyes, too, and knew that we knew. The bluff was up. "Okay, everybody, this is a raid," he said, and flashed a badge. "You're all under arrest for being on premises used for prostitution."

As if on cue, the front door opened, and in walked the big plainclothes policeman I recognized as the one they call Scarface. "Good evening, Miss Hollander," he said, leering at me. "I told you we would get you again."

Eight uniformed cops stormed through the front door and started turning the place over like a pancake. But the scene that followed was more like a Keystone comedy than an efficient police raid.

Bureaus were turned inside out, and men started loading everything that wasn't nailed down onto a cart. My childhood love letters, family photo albums, and even my collection of cookbooks were stuffed aboard. "Let me have those back?" I asked the cop standing guard over the cart, "unless you plan on making some delicious Dutch pea soup down at the station." What'd he do? He shook his head, and refused to release my cookbooks.

Booze that I had bought from a customer, trading one girl for one case, was taken. Cigarettes bought duty-free in the Dutch islands were also taken. None of this worried me. What *was* worrying me were my valuable black book of customer listings and cash book standing on an open shelf. The last time the police took these, I had to buy them back under the table. This time I decided to steal them back.

The cop guarding the cart looked like a horny guy (and men are always men), so I pulled out a collection of pornographic pictures from a drawer. "Hey, look at these," I said, handing him the pictures. In a minute or two, this ape gets so juiced up he calls the others over. And they obliged by gathering around the pictures, soon making obscene comments about them. But I certainly didn't mind, because this allowed me to take a few steps behind them and remove my customer book and cash records from the shelf.

I managed to quickly throw the book of names into a hall closet under an empty carton, and from the cash book I tore out all the pages recording my business affairs and then threw it on the cart to avert suspicion. Since nobody was bothering me, I was able to slip into my bedroom, where I stuffed the pages under the wall-to-wall bedroom rug—which I always leave untacked in one corner. I also slid one thousand dollars in cash under the rug, because if those hyenas find money, they usually say there was none and keep it.

Just then a big cop came out of the bedroom with a packet of cigarette papers in one hand. "Okay, where do you keep the pot? We know you have some."

"I don't have any in the house," I lied. "I never use drugs." As he disappeared into the bedroom, I whisked the plastic bag of marijuana out of the hall closet, rushed into the bathroom, and emptied it down the toilet.

Nobody was watching the bathroom, so I went back and forth like a kidney patient getting rid of damning evidence.

Then I saw a uniformed cop who was trying to act as though he were working go to the hall closet with a flashlight. He began going through things and was getting dangerously close to the carton that concealed the big black book.

"Excuse me, sir," I said, and gently shoved him away from the open door, "my mirror is inside this door, and I have to fix my hair." The cop walked back into the bedroom, where his partners were now congregated, looking for pot.

As nobody was guarding the front door, two of the girls and the maid decided to split.

"Okay, everybody, let's go," a big detective said, coming out of the bedroom. He did a head count and found that three girls were missing.

"Where are those cunts?" he asked, with his hand raised, threatening to strike me. "I'll break their fucking legs when I find them."

"I have no idea where they could be," I said evenly. The girls had strolled to freedom via the front door, and had calmly ridden the elevator to safety.

The police arrested everyone, including poor Calvin, and took everyone but me down to the Seventeenth Precinct. I was left alone in my apartment with the three plainclothesmen who first raided my place. The phones kept ringing—customers wanting to come over. The cops answered all the calls and made rough jokes. That would be the last time those johns called me.

My house was a mess, yet they overlooked my goody bag. I was lucky not to have to replace it. Those leg irons and hand-cuffs so carefully collected, and the rare cat-o'-nine-tails the masochists love to feel bite their flesh. My slaves were saved.

The boys from the precinct had a ball cutting all my tele-phone wires: four telephones in my bedroom, four in the living room. Finally they took me down to the station house. But not before I went into the bedroom and got the money I'd hidden. It was about three in the morning when I joined the others being fingerprinted. The newspaper reporters were milling around outside the station house.

It would be a fine story for the sensation-hungry press. Seven girls, six men arrested.

At the station house, the policemen gave us coffee and doughnuts. They let us lie down on tables and get a little sleep, and even switched off the glaring fluorescent lights on the ceil-ing. Calvin was lying beside Aurora, who'd been his date, on one table. She used her big pocketbook for a pillow. Calvin was still being a sweet pussycat, not giving anyone trouble, but that bas-tard lieutenant *had* to give his name out to the press. Calvin is the president of a big company in the Midwest. I can imagine what he thinks of Fun City now. A family, a career, ruined for half an hour of pleasure.

Takis and I were lying beside each other on another table, my head on his shoulder. And now I was horny, by God, was I ever horny. What is the matter with me?

Takis grew a nice hard-on, and I caressed him when I thought nobody was looking. But why give a damn anyway? They couldn't arrest us again.

In a few hours we woke up stiff and tired. The police had a tel-evision set turned on to the morning news. They brought us more coffee and doughnuts. We watched, and there were the girls walking out of my house. Everyone's name on television. "Madam Xaviera's house was raided last night. She was considered to be the queen of the call girls and exchanged girls and customers all over Europe." Wow! At least they made me look good.

At eight o'clock, after the morning news, we were told we would be taken to the Tombs and warned that there were reporters waiting outside. We all wanted to disguise ourselves somehow. Flavia painted a big black moustache under her nose with an eyebrow pencil, put her hair up with a rubber band, and put on her head a civilian porkpie hat she had managed to lift from one of the policemen.

I put glasses on, my hair up, and wore another man's hat we took. Calvin had the best disguise. I gave him my light summer dress I had stuffed in my bag before the cops took me away. He wrapped the dress around his head, making a turban of it, and pulled the end into a veil around his nose and mouth like an Arab *yashmak.*

We walked down the steps of the station house holding newspapers in front of us and stepped into the van which would take us downtown to the Tombs, one of New York City's jails. There can be no atmosphere in any jail in the country as depressing and sordid as at the Tombs.

As we were rudely pushed along the narrow gray hall of the prison toward our cell block, we passed a cell full of transvestites, mostly grotesque gargoyles making pathetic attempts to be what they were not, although a few succeeded *brilliantly.* *Mundus vult decipi decipiatur ergo*, "the world wants to be cheated, so cheat."

Now, after the pleasant stay at the Tombs, I am at Riker's Island. Two years ago jail was as foreign to me as the far side of the moon. Now one more trip here, and I'll know the graffiti on the slime-covered walls by heart.

Two years ago my house was a pleasure retreat you went home to. Now it is a place you drag around, the way a tortoise carries its shell, from precinct to new precinct after each bust. Yes, I am happy in my business and love it. Indeed, some of the happiest moments of my life have happened in the two years I have been rising in the ranks of New York City prostitution to become the biggest and most important madam in town. But why the harassment from police, the heavy bail and fines, the high lawyers' fees, the payoffs? Whom are we bothering? And, as I think about it, I realize that a safe little secretary can save almost as much as I did this last year.

Finally Larry comes with the money. My lawyer, I find, has been outside for three hours, waiting for the money to bail me out. My savings add up to much less than a secretary could save. But I am out again, riding with Larry back to the city. Now I will have to start again.

I smile sort of hopelessly as Larry parks in front of my apartment building. But I'll get a new place, let my customers know where to find me, get my girls together again, and keep giving pleasure to men and women. I can't help myself. To tell you the truth, I am very happy in the business.

Two

A Family Affair

Don't think of me as a poor little girl gone astray because of a misguided or underprivileged childhood. The contrary is true. I come from a very good background and grew up in a loving family atmosphere.

I was born in Indonesia and later received a fine European education. Between my parents and myself, we speak a total of twelve languages—I personally speak five fluently.

Mother, a stately blonde of German and French extraction, was serious-minded but warm and utterly devoted to her family. She was my doctor-father's second wife. His first wife, a White Russian ballerina, had left Indonesia with their only daughter immediately after their divorce. His marriage with my mother was a happy one, even though they were opposites in personality and temperament. There was never any question that he loved only my mother, despite a twinkling eye for a pretty girl.

My father, whom I idolized, was a rare human being—an intellectual, raconteur, lover of the arts, bon vivant, and a truly generous-spirited man. At the height of his highly successful medical career, he owned a large hospital in the then Dutch East Indies, and I later learned that we had two palatial homes, one in Soerabaja and the other in the hill resort area of Bandung, both run by many servants.

But we lost all that when the Japanese invaded the islands and threw my parents and their newborn baby—that is, me—into a concentration camp.

For the three years of the Japanese occupation, my father suffered extreme hardship and torture at the hands of our captors. His crime was not only that he was Dutch but that he was Jewish as well. And this is something few people realize, that the Japanese in Southeast Asia were as anti-Semitic as the Germans in Europe.

The compound we were incarcerated in had a big sign nailed up with the lettering Banksa Jehudi, which was Malaysian for "Jewish Folks."

My mother suffered torture as well, even though she was not Jewish, but because she committed the crime of being married to a Jew. She was once thrown into a little wooden hut full of corpses, where the temperature was like that of an oven, for a week, because she had become hysterical and demanded extra rations of rice and water when I was very sick with fever and dysentery.

My father was sometimes hung by his wrists from a tree with his feet an inch off the ground in the scorching tropical sun. Probably the only reason they didn't let him die was because they needed his medical skills. They finally dragged him away from us to a separate compound, where he was appointed camp doctor for over two hundred women and children. In wartime this can be a kind of living torture, too, especially for a man who hates to see human suffering.

He later told us that he almost went insane during this period worrying about the well-being of his wife and child. And, ironically enough, the first time he *did* see me again was not as a father but as a doctor. This was two and a half years after he'd been taken away.

He had been confined in the men's camp; my mother and I, in a camp for women. After three years my mother and I were released, and we went to the house of Tania, a friend of my parents, half-Russian and half-Indonesian. When they were separated, my mother and father promised that if they survived, they would meet in Soerabaja at Tania's beautiful house with its huge garden.

One day, playing in that garden, I was chasing a bird when I tripped and gashed myself, deep within my buttocks and close to my vagina, on a sharp tree branch. My mother was out, so our *baboe*, a native maid, carried me in her arms to the nearest internment camp, which, in the event of an emergency, the Japanese sometimes allowed us to enter for medical attention. With tears running down my cheeks, I was taken into a cell where my wound was tended by a gentle, dark man. My crying ceased, and I can still dimly remember the touch of his hands.

A few weeks later, the war came to an end, and the men were at last freed. We waited at Tania's, and I was pedaling my tricycle, when my father came up the path. My mother ran to meet him, but he stopped in his tracks, staring at me.

"Good God!" he cried. "Is it possible? That sweet, little child whom I treated, she was my own, darling daughter, my Xaviera!"

When the war ended, our family was finally reunited, although stripped of all our money and possessions, and we went back to Amsterdam to start all over again. My father was already in his forties, but he was not only a man of great moral strength and courage, but also gifted with a capacity for hard work, and with the help of some financial aid from the Dutch government, he soon built up a fine new practice.

In time he acquired such a widespread reputation as a physician that patients came to him from all over Europe. But he never again achieved his former financial status, and I don't think he really much cared about it. He was not the sort of man who was meant to be a millionaire. He was dedicated to medicine and was infinitely more interested in his patients than money. Some of them were more important to him than his own family. I even knew him to postpone our vacation if a patient needed him. Whatever the hour, he tended to his patients' needs, and sometimes to my mother's distress. Especially if the patient was an attractive woman with nothing more wrong with her than an imaginary stomachache. And a yen for my father.

One of my father's patients was a voluptuous sexpot of a woman, about twenty-four, whom my mother and I called the mustard girl simply because she worked in a mustard factory.

He was treating her primarily for asthma but also—as my mother later found out—for hyperactive sexual urges. Evidently my father's small affair with the mustard girl came to my mother's attention when she saw a mink coat listed in his office accounts. Not very smart of him.

From then on, shortly after the mustard girl came for her visit, which was always after work in the evenings, my mother usually found some excuse to walk into my father's office— which was attached to our home.

One evening Mother and I were in the kitchen putting away the dishes at a time when the mustard girl was having her "treatments," and Mother quietly said, "I think I will take a cup of coffee in to your father." She poured it into his favorite mug and went to his office. Suddenly there was such a commotion I thought the Zuider Zee had burst through the dike. There was yelling and screaming, doors opening and slamming, and china breaking. And with some reason. My mother had walked in unannounced and found the mustard girl, her mink coat open and nothing on underneath, down on her knees lustily sucking my father's penis.

She grabbed my father's patient by the hair and threw her out into the snow, minus shoes and stockings or anything but that precious mink coat. En route, my mother forbade the mustard girl ever to walk through our door again.

My father had retreated into the house, and so Mother then picked up most of our good china and hurled it at my father's head. By this time *I* had retreated to the top of the staircase, where I stood ready to try to intervene if there was going to be a bloodbath. But instead Mother ordered Father out of the house and threatened him with divorce.

My father, as I have stated, was a man of unusual courage. Throughout all the savage things which happened to him during the war, I doubt he shed a tear. But this night he wept openly, because he did love my mother very much and realized how much he had hurt her over a harmless bit of nonsense with an easy piece like the mustard girl.

I was only eleven at the time, but despite my age I could understand that the whole event was not to be taken really seriously. I already recognized that sex and love could mean two different things to two different people. For Father, the mustard girl had been sex—or satisfying a passing appetite. For my mother, his was deep, undying love.

My mother, with her intense German pride, was madly jealous of my father, who was a real Don Juan. Although he was fifteen years older than she, he had a youthful charm, and she could usually sense when something was going on behind her back. As a doctor making his rounds, my father met plenty of temptations to fool around.

So, as a young child, I would often creep out of bed and listen at the top of the stairs to them quarreling. My mother would always be the one to start, and as their voices rose, she would deluge him with recriminations. It was not till I was in my teens that I discovered that although sex and love often went together, they certainly were not the same thing.

But, generally, the atmosphere in our home was warm and loving, and there was never any taboo on sex or nudity. I was used to seeing my father hug my mother in the bathroom, or come to think of it, anywhere in the house. I felt an intense excitement, deep inside me, when I watched his hands roam over her tall, slender body and fondle her breasts. They would kiss in front of me, and at any time of the day, might disappear for hours into their bedroom.

So, even when I was quite young, I had a fair idea of what went on between adults, and how my parents' disputes would be smoothed over in bed. My mother used to tell me, when I was a bit older, that the secret of a successful marriage was to sleep in a double bed. However, before I reached that stage of awareness, I was curious of what exactly took place when their bedsprings were merrily squeaking, and I would sneak out of my room and tiptoe into theirs, which was next to mine. The wild motion of their sheets would suddenly stop, and I would plead to be allowed to sleep in between them, because I had a nightmare or felt lonely or for any other excuse which I would dream up. My father was often reluctant, since he would be left hanging (or perhaps it would be more correct to say, left standing). I loved to press my belly against my mother's buttocks. Her body was always warm and had a fresh, feminine aroma, and as I clasped her full, firm breasts, I would relish the smoothness of her skin. How different from the prickly hair of my father's chest and his muscular body, which fascinated me and so aroused my curiosity that I would peep under the sheets at the way his penis stood erect before he awoke in the morning!

As I grew older, I became more and more attached to my father, and my ambition was to be as intelligent and respected as he was throughout his life. Freud was dead right in my case: if I were to meet a man who reminded me of my father, I would doubtless fall madly in love with him. I was an only child and hopelessly spoiled, not merely in the things I was given, but above all, by the constant devotion which was lavished on me by my parents. My father guided my mental development like the Professor Henry Higgins of *My Fair Lady* and saw to it that my talent for foreign languages was fully cultivated. He encouraged me to study Greek, Latin, French, and German in high school and made it a rule that on weekends, in the summer at the beach or in the winter in the country house, we all conversed in nothing other than a foreign tongue.

On Saturday it would be, say, French or German, and the next day perhaps English. Each year as well we would spend at least one month's vacation in a foreign country so I could improve my accent or else begin to learn another language—say, Spanish or Italian. It was an extraordinary education.

On the other hand, until I was twenty-one I always went on vacation with my parents, unlike most of my friends, who went in unchaperoned groups, because my mother treated me like her little chicken and did not want me exposed to moral danger.

"Keep your virginity until you're married, Xaviera," I remember her saying. "I was a virgin when I got married, and that is how every girl should be. Then your husband will never be able to throw your past up in your face or call you a whore. You will be able to walk with your head high, and nobody can ever say bad things about you." Which all seemed pretty old-fashioned, considering the education in relaxed nudity I was getting at home.

These days you would have to walk around like a Diogenes— armed with a lantern and looking for an honest man—to find a virgin over sixteen.

Anyway, for the time being she did not have to worry about me, because the person I was in love with could never take my virginity. Her name was Helga.

Helga was my closest friend at high school, and for the past year I had nursed a flaming desire for her and did not know why. I vaguely knew about lesbians, but I did not connect myself with those half-man, half-woman types with short hair and long pants that my older schoolmates, giggling, pointed out in the streets.

Helga never returned my feelings, and indeed she did not know lesbians existed, except that she may have wondered why I was always accidentally bumping into her beautiful boobs.

Helga was sixteen, one year older than me, and we were like sisters sharing all our girlhood secrets. But as sexually precocious as I instinctively was, she was just as sweet and innocent.

By fifteen I had already kissed my boyfriend with my tongue, explored his body all over, and had even sucked his cock. Helga never knew about this, but she was aware that I was a little more educated in this direction than she was.

One day my beloved Helga turned to me for the benefit of my advanced knowledge about such things.

"Xaviera, I have something quite embarrassing to ask you," she began shyly as we sat in the recreation room during lunch hour. "And I need your help . . . Tonight Peter Korver has asked me to a party, and I am afraid he is going to want a good-night kiss."

Weirdly enough, when she told me her date that night was with a boy who was one of the most sought-after catches in high school, I was jealous, not of her, but of him.

"You'll never believe this," she went on, "but I have never ever kissed a boy in my life, and I don't know how to react."

I was surprised at her absolute virtue, because she was definitely one of the best-looking girls in the school. She was tall, slim, big-boobed, and had a mass of silky dark hair cascading around her beautiful face.

"Could you explain what I should do?" she asked.

"Of course, Helga," I said. "Let's go over to your place after school, and I'll teach you."

It was wintertime and thus dark at four o'clock when school let out. We doubled up on my bicycle and rode over to her house.

I chained the bicycle to a rail, and we entered the darkened hallway, which I decided would be a perfect setting for the scene, because Helga was from a religious, conservative family who would hardly take kindly to their daughter exchanging romantic gropes with a girlfriend in her bedroom.

I suggested we creep into the cavernlike area under the stairs from the foyer to the second floor of the apartment building, because "this is probably where you and Peter will be when he wants to kiss you."

I coaxed her gently against the hallway wall, and there, under the heavy oak staircase, started making love to my girl.

Helga was submissive at first, although I believe she expected something a little less realistic than *I* had in mind.

"Let me hold you the way a man usually holds a girl," I began, and slipped one arm around her waist and the other around her shoulder. Then I took her chin softly in my hand and planted a kiss on her lips. She stood there stiffly with her eyes and her mouth closed.

"Open your lips, Helga," I urged. "*Nobody* kisses with them closed." She obediently parted her lovely mouth, and I eased my tongue inside. At first she tightened and drew away. "Relax," I whispered; "this is what everybody does, and it is the only way you will learn." My pink serpent of a tongue was exploring her mouth, and I lingered for a passionate eternity until she became restless.

"Now give me yours," I said, and as her sweet-tasting tongue entered my mouth, I thought I would go insane with excitement. I wished the moment could proceed in slow motion, but if I took too much time, she might become impatient or suspicious and walk away.

"No kiss is complete without some attention to the neck and shoulders," I said next, and I started kissing her ears and her neck and pulling back her sweater to get to her breast.

Not really knowing what was happening to her pent-up adolescent sexuality, she was getting carried away. She threw her head back to reveal a pale, slender neck, and goose bumps came out on her flesh.

At that moment the front door opened, and a tenant, accompanied by an icy wind, walked past us and vanished along the hall. I pressed Helga to the wall in a protective gesture. She relaxed and responded.

"After kissing, you have to know how to caress and be caressed," my instruction continued, and I unbuttoned the coat she wore over a sweater and skirt. Then I slid one hand under her sweater, into her bra, and cupped one of her breasts. My other hand went under my own skirt, and I started stroking myself.

I got so frantically excited that I would have loved to have been a man with a big penis and put it inside her. But all I had was a hardened little clitoris.

While she was in her slightly dazed state, I moved my mouth down under her sweater and started sucking those glorious breasts with the erect nipples. As I did so, I also took one of her long legs and pulled it up underneath my skirt between my legs; then I rubbed faster and faster till stars exploded in my head and I fell off the earth.

I was breathless—and Helga was shocked. She had asked how to respond like a lady to an innocent first kiss and had just been seduced in the hallway by a love-crazed schoolgirl. She mumbled something or other and hastily ran up the stairs.

For the next few weeks I was lovestruck and unhappy and followed her everywhere like an adoring puppy, praying for a chance once more to get my hands on her gorgeous body. If she played tennis, I played tennis; if she went horseback riding, so did I; and when she joined the snooty rowing club, I joined the snooty rowing club, just so that I could catch a glimpse of her.

I would love to watch her sliding back and forth on the bench of the boat in her shorts, and would follow her to the shower afterward and wish I could rub the soap all over her magnificent body as she stood there wearing nothing else but a bathing cap.

As Helga matured a little, she started to recognize my absolute infatuation and began teasing me, which would drive me more and more out of my mind, and for two whole years I walked around adoring and desiring her, even after I lost my virginity to a boy at the age of seventeen.

The loss of virginity was for most girls a turning point in their lives; for me it was a mere technicality. For two years, with Dennis, a student at the same high school as myself and a couple of years older than me, we had kissed, cuddled, fingered, and fondled among the sand dunes or behind the bushes in the park. We had even carried out certain oral activities on each other's genitals, but without much expertise. His sperm had splashed over my breasts, in my hair, and in my pubic hair, but never inside me.

The day arrived when we decided that we would go all the way. After all, what was the point of that stupid hymen, although Mummy wanted me to get married as a virgin? It was odd that, with my liberated family background, she should have this obsession with "purity." Now, we had been children long enough, and when kind friends offered us the use of their apartment, and their bed, the time had arrived for us to become adults. Up to now, Dennis had penetrated me for no more than an inch or so, but each time he got deeper, and I would move back, so that my hymen had been stretched like an elastic band.

There was no cracking or snapping or blood and pain, just a sensation, warm, good, and intense, as his penis at last slipped inside my eager pussy. Although he was big and thick, he did not hurt me, but it seemed as if his cock became mine and he possessed my cunt, as he moved faster and deeper inside me, and our bodies melted together. Each time he pulled back, I pressed him further into me, until with a joyful scream, he shot his load for the very first time inside my pussy, and I came instantly, biting his lip hard in my excitement. I was seventeen, and at last, a real woman, warm, wet, and willing for more!

Far more significantly, I must confess that from the moment I lost my virginity I became absolutely wild about sex, and even threw over my steady boyfriend in pursuit of it. I couldn't care less who I did it with, even my relatives. In fact, the idea of sampling forbidden fruit made incest all the more exciting. The only taboo against it was don't make babies, that's all.

In my early teens when I first heard the facts of life from older friends, I used to wish I had a big brother so I could fuck him. In my late teens I did gratify my taste for forbidden fruit and actually made it with some members of my family. And not by accident.

My first attempt was my mother's brother, my favorite uncle, who adored me as a child in a paternal way and as an adolescent in what was definitely a more carnal way.

One weekend when my family took me with them to visit his family in Düsseldorf, Germany, we made an assignation to sneak away to a motel room and make love. But the prospect of the clandestine affair apparently so excited him that his wife was able to guess what he was up to. She did not let him out of her sight until my family and I returned to Amsterdam, so the whole endeavor was aborted.

The second family affair was more successful, and it happened a few years later with the twenty-eight-year-old son of another uncle, who had come to stay with our family and see the sights of Holland. He was a big, strapping young German, and certainly no virgin.

It was my job to take him out and show him the town, and I was even allowed to stay out past my midnight curfew because he was a relative. The first night I showed him the regular tourist sights and sent him home early. The second night I showed him the fun spots like the "girls in the windows" in Amsterdam's legalized red-light district on the canals, then took him back to his hotel and seduced him. He was not bad, nothing special, a typical strong German, but with an unromantic soul.

By this time, I had graduated from high school with top marks, studied music for a year, and then gone to work for one of Amsterdam's leading ad agencies as an assistant account executive.

From the moment I began work, I approached my job with the large amount of enthusiasm and dedication with which I have done everything else in my life—and still do today. The work was nice, but it didn't have what you call in America immediate "upward mobility," so I decided to try for something else. Even in those early days I had the desire and the drive to be Numero Uno. I'd heard that the Manpower Employment Agency was conducting a contest for the best multilingual secretary in Holland, and being competitive and ambitious, I decided to enter it.

The contest was to be judged on best typing, shorthand in four languages, translating skills, poise, and personality. There were several exams leading to the final, which required each entrant to write a two-hundred-word poem as a publicity pamphlet for the employment agency. I was the youngest of the sixty contestants—and, as it happened, the most successful. I won the title of Best Secretary in Holland.

Television interviews, newspaper articles, and a trip to England, as well as $1,000 prize money, followed, and I was appointed a unit head at Manpower—a job that was, coincidentally, not unlike the one I do today. I became a true "matchmaker." Now, a banker might call up the agency for the services of a secretary or a typist. Later in my career, I would be called by a businessman who wanted to be provided with a blonde, brunette, or redhead. It all came down to demand and supply. That was when I discovered my best skills were administrative, in an intermediary capacity. I also learned another valuable lesson from that job: that if you have real initiative, it is best to work as an independent if you can, because others tend to sit back and reap the profits of your hard efforts.

For relaxation after a hectic week, I would go with friends on weekends to a white-sand beach resort not far from Amsterdam named Zandvoort. This beautiful beach stretched along the entire Dutch coastline and had little terraced cabanas and gaily decorated restaurants where you could sit out front and have meals and refreshments. Each restaurant had a name and a number, so when you wanted to make a date with someone, you would say, "See you later at Wilhelmina's number twenty-four."

One weekend I went to Zandvoort with a drummer friend named Kuuk, and we both had a brand-new personal experience—we discovered Seaview number twenty-two, and the colorful and gay crowd that hung out there.

Most men were fashionably dressed in minuscule bikinis which hardly covered their emphasized assets, designer T-shirts, and Pucci or St. Laurent scarves. There were also lots of well-groomed poodles jumping around that belonged to the gay boys.

The girls, as I soon found out, were predominantly gay as well.

The only really straight person there was my friend Kuuk. Extremely handsome and well built, he had all the gay boys swarming over him.

Left alone, I introduced myself all around until I came upon a woman whose face seemed strangely familiar, although as far as I was aware I didn't have any dyke friends.

"Hi," the pretty red-haired girl said to me; "how have you been these last few years?"

"Me? Are you sure you mean me?"

"Yes, you little 'butch,'" she said, laughing.

"What do you mean by that?" I asked her.

"My name is Betty. I was your teacher in high school, and I used to see you lusting after Helga at the same time *I* was dying to have an affair with you."

Betty, who taught us art and designing, was not exactly what you could call a schoolmarm type. She was always dressed in elegant pantsuits and had told us she was engaged to the country's top actor. Still, I was informed enough to know her fiancé was definitely gay, but I never imagined that for her part she was a lesbian.

"I could tell you were a little 'butch' in those days," she volunteered. I was surprised to hear that. I may have been strong and well built, and I had shortish blond hair, too, but when I look back at pictures taken in those days, I would say I looked like the average attractive, but sporty, schoolgirl.

Betty now took my arm. Pupil and former teacher went around and talked to all the lesbians. And from this time on I willingly got into the female homosexual scene.

One day, Betty sent to the Manpower office where I worked a girlfriend who was obviously looking for more than just a job. Elsbeth had blond, curly hair reaching right down to her shoulders and a lithe, athletic body. Her low-cut summer dress left nothing to the imagination. She looked very feminine, and I was content that my getting her a temporary post led to a romance between us. However, our affair did not last long. She discarded her pretty clothes and took to wearing more and more masculine gear, ending with blue jeans and a sloppy sweater or a cowboy shirt. Also, she started to drink and smoke heavily, and her butchness turned me off, so that after a couple of months I gave up seeing her. Actually, she had never given me a proper orgasm because she always wanted to use some gadget, such as a dildo or a vibrator, which I did not want in case I got hooked on them. She never even sucked me off: I guess oral sex was not much done in those days even among lesbians, and I was never keen on fingering, because I am very sensitive.

At that time I didn't smoke or drink because of a truly sincere agreement I had made with my parents while a teenager. They had said that if I didn't drink or smoke until I was eighteen they would buy me a motor scooter, and at eighteen they promised me a car if I could abstain from both these things until I was twenty-one. I got both the scooter and the car and, astonishingly enough, to this day have never taken an alcoholic drink or normal cigarette.

Elsbeth, the little dyke, was madly in love with me and considered herself my male partner, but as I got more into the lesbian activity, I discovered I was definitely the dominant type, and so we had a "supremacy" fight and broke up.

I met many more girlfriends through my female hairdresser, who was also Betty's lover, and my sex life soon became part heterosexual and part homosexual, and sometimes a happy mixture of both.

It was also around this time that I was taken under the wing of a sophisticated older couple who lived in a magnificent seventeenth-century house in the artists colony on Amsterdam's Prinsen Island. Daedo, the husband, was a man of forty-two, and Sylvia, his wife, was eight years older. Nights and weekends I would often sleep over and spend a lot of time gossiping with Sylvia, an attractive, vivacious woman, while Daedo, who owned an advertising agency, worked in his study.

One evening, Sylvia phoned and asked me to hurry over to her house. I jumped on my scooter, but when I arrived, the place seemed to be deserted. Then I noticed a few oil lamps faintly flickering, and her dog began to bark. I went in and, since she had complained of a bad backache and asked me to give her a massage, made my way upstairs to where I presumed her bedroom was. There was the sound of water running in the bathroom, and suddenly I was confronted by the sight of Sylvia, superb in her nakedness, slowly and languorously soaping herself and smiling at me.

"Come inside, Xaviera," she called. "Get out of those clothes and join me."

For a moment I hesitated, and then I slipped off my dress and panties. Sylvia seemed so self-assured and experienced that I suffered a pang of shyness, but I climbed into the shower, and she started to rub soap onto my back in loving, sensual movements. Once we were dry, we went into her bedroom, and she asked me to give her a massage. She was still naked, but I had put on my panties. I sat astride her, and with firm, strong movements worked on her back, in the way my father had taught me. Sylvia began to moan softly from pleasure, and I realized that my panties were nice and moist. I guess she must have noticed too, for all at once, she turned around, pulled me close, and covered my face and neck with kisses. Her fingers lightly scratched my back, and I was getting very turned on and so confused that I hardly noticed when she pulled off my panties.

I let my own fingers stroke her lovely, pale body, and she pushed my head toward her breast. I took those big, dark nipples hungrily and sucked on them as if I were a baby.

"Xaviera, darling, how about kissing me just a bit lower?" she coaxed, and guided me toward her navel.

Her soft, white belly quivered every time I touched a sensitive spot, and I heard her gasp as I moved purposefully down to her triangle. Never before had my lips approached any woman's vagina, not even during my encounter with the girl I had found a job for at Manpower, and I was just getting acquainted with her pussy when I heard somebody quietly enter the room. I was ready to jump up and get dressed, but Sylvia pushed my head back into her lap and told me to get on with what I had been doing. I could hear Daedo pulling off his shoes and softly sliding them under the bed. Then his warm body was next to mine, under the sheets. Raising myself onto my knees, I could not resist taking his stiff prick between my breasts and, leaning forward, ran my tongue along his shaft right up to the scrotum. Daedo had to hold himself back from coming, and he wriggled until he was able to bring his mouth to satisfy my avid cunt, where his lips soon found my swollen labia. Sylvia, meanwhile, was masturbating and thoroughly enjoying the scene, and occasionally giving me gentle bites on the back, which brought me out in goose bumps. Finally, I mounted Sylvia, pushing my legs between hers, while Daedo, supporting himself on his elbows and knees, climbed on top of me. He thrust his hard cock into my pussy from behind, while I rubbed my Venus hill against Sylvia's cunt, and the three of us came in a great, simultaneous orgasm, which was quite an acrobatic performance. Their little dog stood at the bedside, wagging his tail in amazement. I could not help thinking that Sylvia's bad back had received unorthodox treatment and that maybe it had just been an excuse to lure me into their sex-nest, but who was complaining?

This turned out to be the first of many threesomes; in fact, we became firm fucking friends. One evening, we were in a crazy mood, and Daedo put on an act as a waiter, balancing a lighted candle in a candlestick on his cock and carrying a glass of orange juice in each hand as he came into the bedroom, stark naked but with a napkin over his arm.

But after a couple more months, I had pretty much had it with Holland. Apart from a few liberated friends like Sylvia and Daedo, I found the people too solemn and puritanical for my liking. I was lucky enough to be living in Amsterdam, the capital. God knows what it would have been like in some remote village! I would rather have died than sat about, bored out of my skull, with nothing better to do than to gaze at the cows grazing in the fields.

And when it came to romance, the Dutch were not renowned as fiery lovers, nor for their inventiveness in bed. As soon as I was "going steady" with some guy, he wanted to get engaged, and that was a prospect which scared the life out of me. I was too young to settle down and get married, but the proposals kept coming, and when my would-be partner for life started talking about what we would need in the home—pressure cooker, cutlery, linen, etc.—I knew that it was time to split again.

Friends of mine who had visited me recently, just arriving from South Africa, had told me about the beauty of this country, and the warm year-round climate. In case I would be interested in immigrating there, the South African government would pay the airfare completely. So . . . away from cold and misery and rainy summers. Down to the sun and my sister, who lived there as well. In fact, I was getting a bit bored with the Dutch mentality, even though Holland is a very charming country and Amsterdam lately has become one of the swingingest cities in Europe. Maybe it was not so much Holland itself, but my inner hunger for someplace new and exciting. The fact that I had my stepsister (a daughter from my father's first marriage) living in Johannesburg with her husband and children made it more encouraging for me to go there.

When I decide to do something, I do it quickly and efficiently. I arranged visas, booked my ticket, and organized my private life to leave Holland.

There was only one last thing to do before boarding the plane. I had to say good-bye to my lovely Helga, who was now eight and one half months pregnant.

When I went to see her for the last time, she was standing there in a nightie, and nothing was more exciting to me than to see that big belly sticking out, and those beautiful breasts.

"Helga," I said, "please let me touch your belly and suck your nipples, because they are more beautiful than ever."

She hesitated at first, now not because of modesty but because her husband, whom I could not stand, might walk in. He didn't care much for me, and the feeling was mutual. Maybe it was jealousy, but I found him a real bore.

His name was De Boer, which means farmer, and it suited him perfectly. He had already gone into her mail and found the love letters I sent her from all over Europe. Looking back, I guess she thought I was simply foolish, because she never even replied. However, on this last visit, she agreed to let me have my wish and touch her, and she lifted up her nightie.

I gently lowered my mouth around the nipples, and a trace of milk escaped, and the loving feeling was still there, and ever since I have ardently admired pregnant women.

I couldn't believe that after five years I was finally sucking and caressing those divine breasts, and Helga was letting me. In all the experience and sex I have had in the intervening time, this is still the most precious moment I can remember.

I think I was just about to tell her how I loved her, when a red-faced and furious De Boer stormed in and ordered me out of his house.

"If I ever catch her here again, I'll throw you both out!" he screamed at his wife.

A few days later my family and friends bade me a tearful farewell on my flight to South Africa, and everyone was crying, including me.

"Come back to us," my mother said through her tears, but even then I knew I never would, at least not for a long time.

The only thing that tied me to Holland besides my parents, believe it or not, was Helga, and that was an impossible dream.

Three

South Africa

The flight from Amsterdam to Johannesburg promised to be very long but not necessarily dull. I was seated alongside an attractive Italian businessman with a divine sense of humor and a cultured manner. During dinner, served immediately after takeoff, we enjoyed a spirited conversation, discovering we shared a mutual interest in classical music, among other things.

He was such a charming person that, by the time the stewardess removed our trays, I already wanted to go down on him. A lot of acrobatic skill was required to accomplish this feat without being observed. The way we finally did it was to cover me to the tip of my head with a light blanket while I pretended to be getting my vanity bag from under his window seat. Doing it got us so turned on that we wanted to make love all the way. But first, we had to be patient until the girls handed out blankets and pillows, dimmed the cabin lights, and everyone was settled down.

As soon as the coast was clear we removed the armrests from the seats, squeezed down together under the blanket, he facing my back spoon-fashion, and proceeded to make love. We had to be very quiet, and, we soon discovered, very careful, because a couple of times he became overamorous and I almost fell down between the seats.

We made a game of doing it between the stewardesses walking up the aisle to answer call lights and the passengers walking sleepily to the lavatory. The challenge of making love thirty thousand feet in the air made it even more exciting.

It was rather like sardines in a can, to tell you the truth, and very uncomfortable, but, even so, by the time we flew into daybreak we had managed to make love three times. As breakfast was served, we got up, stiff and sticky, and finally stretched our cramped legs.

The rest of the trip I spent sprucing up to meet my stepsister and her husband, Dan, whom I had seen only once before, and that was when Mona had traced my father down in Amsterdam while she was there from South Africa on her honeymoon.

Like me, Mona was born in Indonesia, but her mother, formerly a beautiful Russian ballerina, took her away from there after the divorce, and she and my father completely lost touch.

At the time I met them, I remember thinking what a lovely person she was and how handsome was her husband. Even as a fourteen-year-old virgin, I had the tingling desire to make love to him someday. Dan was a mining engineer of French Huguenot descent, tall, well built, with dark curly hair. He was a true Afrikaner, stubbornly assertive and proud of his masculinity, and a terrific storyteller.

Both of them were at Johannesburg Airport to meet me, and it was a happy reunion with lots of hugging, kissing, and laughing. Mona was just as dear as I remembered, and Dan was even more handsome.

Also there to meet me was a girl named Deenie, whom I had never met before but had corresponded with through Sylvia. She recognized me from a photo I had sent, and she walked straight over and introduced herself to me and my relatives.

Deenie worked for KLM, the Dutch airline, and we exchanged telephone numbers, agreed to meet when I was settled in, and Mona, Dan, and I set out for my new home.

After a half-hour drive, we arrived at a magnificent two-story house in an exclusive outer suburb of Johannesburg. The building was set in sprawling lawns, which made a vast playground for my niece, eight, and two nephews, seven and six, and two huge dogs, a Great Dane and a German shepherd.

To one side was a luxurious swimming pool, the other a three-car garage, and behind was a chicken farm, Mona's pet project, which she ran with the aid of some of their servants.

Life was easy in the South African sunshine, and the family treated me like royalty. I was not allowed to lift a finger around the house, so the days were spent lazying by the pool, working on my suntan.

But the nights were often empty. In those days there was no television in South Africa because of what people say was a deliberate government policy to contain apartheid. So if they didn't invite a neighbor couple over for dinner, there was little else to do. During the first couple of weeks I would sit in the living room, listening to classical records, being baby-sitter, while my sister and her husband attended some formal dinner or other function. The eerie silence would be punctuated only by the shrill chirp of crickets or an occasional bird, and the only stirring would be when the wind caught the diaphanous curtains.

At these times, the realization I was the only adult in this big lonely house would make me feel melancholy and homesick, and to kill time I wrote long, long letters to my family and friends.

I was also acutely feeling the absence of a strong male body to caress me and, to put it bluntly, satisfy my sexual cravings. In Amsterdam I was used to regular sex at least once a week and twice on weekends with my steady boyfriend, and all of a sudden I was deprived.

The urge to have a lover was really getting to me—forget about masturbation, since that was something I rarely ever did—but there didn't seem to be any unattached males around except for the servants, whom I wouldn't consider quite apart from the fact there is a penalty of nine months' imprisonment in South Africa for crossing that kind of a color line.

One day I was left in charge of the children while their parents went to a morning wedding. I occupied them with games, and then we all took a swim in the pool.

Jonathan, the seven-year-old, seemed to have a prematurely developed sexual instinct, and climbed with his legs around me, somehow undid my bra, and started feeling my breast. As he hung there in the water with his lilliputian legs around me, I felt his penis becoming slightly hard. I had no intention of letting it go any further, so I calmed him down, dried him off, and we all went in to have lunch.

Since this was hardly a very satisfactory kind of love life, I started thinking seriously about finding a place of my own where I could conduct my private activities in a more mature, conventional manner. I also wanted to look for a job, because I was not accustomed to total idleness.

But Mona didn't want me to leave. She loved having a sister around, because, for the first time in her adult life, here was someone to whom she could confide her intimate secrets.

Although I never met Mona's mother, the woman must have been as much like her daughter as I was like my father. As wild and as extroverted as I was, she was shy and introverted.

Mona was a warm, spontaneous person, but strictly raised, and almost on the prudish side. I was amused at the way she wore flannel pajamas that concealed her body from the neck down, even in the hot South African climate, in case one of her children should wander in and really check out her body. At the pool she would even wear a "decent" one-piece bathing suit.

How different it was from my liberal upbringing, when seeing my father with a hard-on was almost as natural as seeing my mother with a hat on.

With the need for mature, conventional sex now critical in my mind, I found myself at home alone one day with my brother-in-law.

We walked over to the swimming pool, and I settled myself on my belly on a towel. In an innocent voice, I asked Dan if he would undo my bra strap, so that I could get a nice, uniform suntan without an ugly, white strip. He was wearing just a pair of khaki slacks, and I liked the look of his great, hairy chest. He was fumbling with my bikini top, and I casually brushed away some ants which were crawling over his feet. There was something provocative in the way I stroked each of his toes, and when he had at last unclasped my bra, I leaned forward, ostensibly to remove the last of the ants which had ventured on to his chest, pressing my breasts against his bare knees and letting my fingers play through his hair and upward to his shoulder blades. He stayed sitting, and by now our bodies were so close that I was virtually in his lap. I had slid my body up, rubbing myself against his flesh, and my tits were poised, firm and inviting, right under his nose.

His glasses had fallen off into the grass, and there was an urgent, hungry look in his eyes when he opened his mouth to taste the sweet fruit which I dangled in front of him. I played hard to get and teased him every time he tried to close his lips around one of my tits. We sprang to our feet, and he must have chased me three times around the pool before I fell on the grass, and he finally succeeded in attaining my breasts, feverishly sucking one nipple while his hands fondled the other. There was no way that he could hide his erection, and it seemed to embarrass him. Holding me tight as if to make sure that I did not melt away, he made his confession.

"Xaviera, I swear that in the eleven years that I have been married to Mona, I have never so much as looked at another woman—that is, until you arrived. But you are a witch, you are driving me crazy. God, I could fuck you here and now beside the pool, and maybe that would set me free! My conscience does not give me a moment's peace, but all the time I have been planning and scheming how I could get you alone. And you being Mona's sister, I know it is not right, but what can I do?"

Such a handsome, square hunk of conservative manhood was exactly what I needed at that moment, and I resolved to overcome his Afrikaner stubbornness. The fact that he had never once cheated on his wife made it all the more exciting. My mouth was watering at the thought that I was going to have him all to myself—and now.

Seducing him presented no problem. My long, sensitive fingers gently scratched all over his body, and my mouth was pretty active as well. His nipples were taut, and the position in which we were lying enabled me to do all sorts of lovely things with my mouth between his thighs completely unobserved, even if anybody should have been looking. I could see that Dannie was struggling with his conscience, but his instincts were gaining the upper hand.

"Sweetheart," I murmured, "let's go inside and get ourselves something cool to drink."

At the foot of the stairs, with glasses of Coca-Cola in our hands, I guided him toward my bedroom. I sat on the bed, topless but still wearing my bikini pants, and his conscience put up its final, hopeless resistance.

"No, no I mustn't," he breathed. "I would never be able to forgive myself, not with my wife's own sister. Xaviera, I want you! I should leave, please let me go."

While he was speaking, I held his belt with one hand and with the other undid the buckle. His objections were getting feebler and feebler, and I made him strip down to his white underpants.

"You must behave," he murmured as he made an unconvincing attempt to push my head away from its exploration within his pants.

"Adorable," I commented as I closed my lips around the tip of his cock.

"Don't do that," he said. His cock was swelling up to double its former size in my mouth, and I enjoyed every inch of it.

He made as if to push me away, but his fingers were caressing my hair, and he was pushing my head deeper into his genitals so frenziedly that I was practically deep-throating him. Suddenly he was driving hard: in a few firm strokes he came in my mouth, and I gulped down his sperm.

Dan was still wearing his jockey shorts, which looked quite ridiculous with his penis at half-mast peeping through the fly, so I pulled them off, and then to be sociable I stepped out of my own bikini pants. Within five minutes, we were passionately making love. However, this time, after an eternity of kissing, it was the turn of Dan's mouth to do the exploring. My room reeked, and my body was soaked with sweat, sperm, and saliva. It will be a long time before I forget the smell and the squishy sound of our amorous movements of that session! I was so excited that the merest touch of his hand or tongue sent me into a whole chain reaction of orgasms, but it was when he penetrated me really hard and deep that we came together in one wild, wonderful peak.

Inevitably, a few minutes later I found Dan in the pangs of guilt and remorse and panicking lest Mona arrived and caught us in the act. Just as inevitably, ten minutes later still, we were at it again, our limbs intertwined and our mouths pressed hard together. But I realized that my brother-in-law was a true beginner in the art of making love and totally unaware that there was any alternative to the missionary position. So I set about giving him some basic instruction on how to please a woman. Mona should have been grateful to me.

He was thrilled when I laid between his legs and sucked him, but when I sensed that he was approaching his climax, I mounted him and rode his rampant cock like an Amazon warrior. Then, without letting him slip out, I turned my body around so that he had a full view of my buttocks. He seemed to be getting the point, since he grabbed my ass while he dug his prick in as far as he could penetrate, and I helped by bending forward and lovingly stroking his feet. His breathing was ragged and his muscles taut as steel, so I knew that he was ready for the grand finale. I jumped off him, crouched on all fours, and got him to take me "doggy" fashion. He did not need much persuading, and I prided myself on the progress of my pupil.

Still we had not finished, and when he had recuperated sufficiently, I lay on the edge of the bed while he took me, standing in front of me and gripping my thighs as if I were a Venus's wheelbarrow! He was really turned on and roared like a lion as he came for the third time. I had lost count of my orgasms; there must have been at least five.

Only then did we realize that the noise outside the house was probably Mona's car pulling up, and Dan scrambled into his clothes to gallop downstairs and meet her as she came in, a picture of nonchalant innocence. Maybe I should have felt guilty, but the release of sexual tension swamped every other emotion.

From that day, Dan and I made all kinds of excuses to get Mona and the kids out of the house. "Why don't you go and play a game of tennis?" "Why don't you take the kids for a drive? Don't you have to deliver some chickens?" he would ask her. My virtuous brother-in-law was turning into an absolute sex maniac. I taught him another ten new positions and made it with him several more times, but then the gravity of what I was doing *did* start to get to me, and I began to feel guilty. I had needed sex, but I also cared for Dan and Mona.

"Listen," I said to him one day, "why don't you go and practice what I've taught you on my sister, too?"

He must have taken my advice, because a week later a new Mona with slightly dark circles under her eyes called me aside and confided in me.

"Xaviera," she began awkwardly, "I think Dan has gone crazy or something; all of a sudden he has become sex hungry . . . And he wants to do it in all different kinds of positions; he even wants me to put my legs over his shoulders. I've never heard of such a thing!"

Of course, her husband's "aberrations" all coincided with the positions I had taught him, and, what's more, she enlisted my aid in figuring out how he had learned them.

"We don't have any sex books in the house, and he can't be having an affair, because he never goes out, so I'm all confused."

"Maybe he's seen some stag films," I said, which was a crazy suggestion, because the South African censorship laws are very strict, and so far as I knew, they had no such thing as blue movies. But I thought I had better offer *some* kind of suggestion.

My guilty conscience began to work by now. I really needed to make love, but just the same, I didn't want to be calculating with my own sister.

Also, I was afraid that if she kept mentioning it to me, I somehow might start laughing and say, "Guess who taught him?"

Either way, it would be better for me, after being there for more than a month, to move out, so I announced that this time I really intended to settle down and get an apartment.

I first went into town and found a good job as an executive secretary with a large advertising agency, and then asked Deenie, the girl from the airport, to help me find an apartment.

She took me to several addresses, and the one I liked best was a spacious one-bedroom place in the Hillbrow section of Johannesburg, the young, swinging heart of the city.

Before I moved out of my sister's house I called Dan aside and gave him a little talk. "Listen," I said, "all this new stuff I taught you is between Mona, you, and me. So please keep it in the family, and don't go out practicing it elsewhere."

The apartment would not be ready until the end of the month, three days away, so Deenie asked me to stay with her.

Her place was smaller than the one I was getting, and it had only one small bed.

The first night I moved in, Deenie surprisingly made no attempt to have any intimacy with me. The second night was curiously the same. By the third night I couldn't stand the sexual tension any longer. "Listen, Deenie," I begged, "please let me make love to you."

That night we had a fantastic time. She was beautiful and exciting and responded to my advances.

For the next two months we had a little affair, but conflict built up again, as in my first lesbian relationship with Elsbeth in Amsterdam. I was more of a butch and liked to please women rather than be pleased. That's why I often give them satisfaction and don't get it myself. Mentally yes, but physically no—for that I need a man.

And that was something else that was missing in a lesbian relationship. Something they can have no way—the real thing, cock. Forget about artificial devices and dildos. I happen to like to fuck, and that is one thing women cannot do with each other, at least not all the way. Emotionally, however, a love affair between two women is sometimes the most beautiful thing on earth, because they have more in common than men and women and more understanding of each other's desires. They are generally less selfish in bed and more gentle.

It didn't take long before I was roaming around looking for male action, and I must say Deenie proved to be very tolerant of me when I did. At times she would come with me after work to a British-style pub called Dawson's, where admen, travel agents, and bankers hung out, and often she picked up a little male something for herself, too. But basically she was a lesbian who specialized, as it were, in seducing older women with turbulent marriages—types who usually treated Deenie very generously and gave her many beautiful presents.

Eventually Deenie and I completely severed our sexual relationship, and I launched on a one-woman sex spree that at one time or another must have included every one of the habitués of Dawson's pub.

I attribute my high libido at the time to the general South African atmosphere. Like any colonial situation where you belong to an overindulged white ruling minority, pampered by servants indentured from the indigenous majority, boredom and irresponsibility inevitably set in.

Apart from our high-salaried, low-taxed jobs, all other energies were channeled into the pursuit of amusement.

The same boring drunks turned up at the same drunken parties, creating an increasingly incestuous circle, with everyone screwing everybody else's wife or girl.

As a consequence of this kind of behavior, so-called standards quickly decline, and the mortality rate on marriages—and human life—increases. For instance, South Africa has one of the highest suicide rates per head of white population in the world.

The figure is also swelled by the number of homosexuals driven over the brink by job, housing, and social discrimination. The gay girls and boys are being chased all over Johannesburg, from one bar to the next, each time their new hangout is raided.

The narrow-minded government—the Afrikaans-speaking people, and *not* the more liberal-minded English—think any form of sex (almost even marital sex) is a sin.

In Jo'burg—or Jewburg, as it is often called because of the overwhelmingly high percentage of Jews who live there—the Afrikaners, old family descendants of the early Dutch colonists, seldom married out of their conservative and cliquey society.

Nevertheless, these apparently stuffy men adored the European girls, freewheeling blond German, Dutch, or Nordic types. They preferred their broad-minded sexual approach, their warmth and spontaneity, and, being the most popular, these girls, myself included, screwed their way around town for free.

At the outset the men would take me to a nice dinner or to the theater, but that gradually dwindled to just bringing around a bottle of wine, and finally, they would just drop by, get laid, and leave.

In no time I acquired quite a reputation in this ofttimes hypocritical crowd, and at parties they would jokingly say, "There goes the flying Dutchman—flying from bed to bed."

It was at this time that I got turned off by the mentality of men. They are basically selfish in their urges, insisting on the right to make love when and how they want it.

Once I tried to extricate myself from the whole rotten web, and they snickered, "What's the matter, has the little nymphomaniac got a disease?"

I did not especially want to be promiscuous, and would have loved a steady boyfriend to share things with and take care of me, but somehow I never met one, and toward the end of this period I was really fed up and depressed by men in general.

My best friends became the male homosexual crowd, who taught me how to cook and appreciate opera and ballet. The only red-blooded male I could confide in during that glum period was a little Jewish photographer named Aubrey. Ours was a platonic relationship, but at least I could depend on him to take me out in the evenings, knowing there was nothing ulterior about his intentions. And it was a barbecue party Aubrey took me to on a November night in 1966 where I met the man I was to become engaged to.

The occasion for the party was Guy Fawkes Day, when the British observe the anniversary of the day a man by that name attempted to blow up their houses of Parliament. It is traditionally celebrated with fireworks, and that is exactly what exploded when I met our host.

Carl Gordon was a twenty-eight-year-old American economist, recently arrived in Johannesburg on a tour of duty for his New York–based management-consulting firm, and he was every woman's idea of the perfect catch.

Carl was extremely good-looking, built like an Adonis, and stylishly dressed in custom-made clothes. He was very virile-looking. On top of that, he lived alone in a fabulous mansion of a house with twin tennis courts and an Olympic-size swimming pool.

"Aubrey"—I nudged my escort—"Carl is the most divine man I have ever seen; how can I get to know him?"

Aubrey was pessimistic. "Don't waste your time, his Greek girlfriend, Elly, sticks to him like glue."

How right he was. From seven o'clock when the party started, until it was about to break up, she watched him like a hawk, and it was only a wicked plot hatched by Aubrey and me—to spike her Irish coffees with triple shots of whiskey—that made her fade from the picture.

Carl, I could sense, was also interested in me, but he barely had time to take down my telephone number and make a tentative date for Sunday, before it was time for everyone to go home.

The rest of the week dragged by. I would sit at my desk during the day or lie in bed at night fantasizing about what a beautiful romance we would have. Sunday could not come fast enough.

The day finally dawned, and I was jolted from my sleep at eight o'clock to answer the jangling phone. But it wasn't Carl. It was Jurgen, a German pilot I had promised weeks before to go horseback riding with that day. There was no wriggling out of it, and even though I loved going to bed with this man, my thoughts were elsewhere that day.

Around five, I insisted he take me home, and just as I inserted my key in my front door, the telephone rang. This time it was Carl.

At six, he arrived at my house, preceded through the door by a huge bunch of red roses with a cute little poem attached saying he had been calling all day and was dying to see me.

That evening I found out Carl was just as I had fantasized him. Intelligent, world traveled, courteous, and considerate. How utterly different from the uncouth run-of-the-mill local male.

Our first date was dinner and dancing at Johannesburg's most fashionable restaurant, and I was so turned on when he held me against his strong chest that my nipples were in constant erection throughout the night. That is as far as it went, though, because I had just started menstruating, and in those days I didn't know how to cope with the situation and would have been acutely embarrassed if he had suggested going to bed.

However, Carl was understanding and didn't push me, and remained as patient as any man could be as we wined and dined together for the next four nights.

By the fifth evening, when both of us were almost clawing the walls, it happened, and it was—as the kids say—like, wow!

Sometimes, when you really dig somebody and for some reason have to resist making love, the beautiful torment of restraint can make the act fantastic when it finally happens.

And it was not that Carl was a very skillful lover. In fact, he was rather inexperienced and came one-two-three. And so did I, because I was so overcome with passion and the desire to have him inside me that I didn't last any longer than he did at first.

Later on I would teach him how to make love properly, just as I have done with almost all of my men—as long as they had the potentials, which include a good body and a strong penis. What also appealed to me was his strong, athletic build and his power of instant recuperation in bed.

And Carl was really huge. Even to this day I have seen only two other men endowed like him. However, generous sexual endowments don't specifically make a man a good lover, but it helps as long as he uses it gently and doesn't crudely bang away, because that can certainly hurt the woman.

With Carl that first night I was lucky I was so turned on and therefore lubricated; otherwise I probably would not have been able to accommodate all of him.

Gradually we became used to each other and each other's bodies, and as our romance progressed, I let it be known to all the old crowd that I was no longer in circulation. "Don't drop by anymore or call me up," I told them all; "I've met my man, and I am in love now."

It would have been more convenient for us both had I moved in with Carl, but we wanted our love affair to get off on the right footing. My mother used to caution me about that.

"Xaviera, I can't blame you if you don't manage to keep your virginity until you are married in these modern times, but try never to live with a man," she said. "You'll give away the best years of your life if you let him have his cake and eat it too and get nothing in return, because a man never marries a woman who allows him to live with her."

Her sentiments seemed quaint at the time, but I was to recall them as being not so old-fashioned, after all.

We moved in a respectable circle of businessmen and their wives, and our affair was indeed on a discreet basis. We respected each other tremendously, and I was very glad he never got to know about my frivolous background. The chances were he never would. Within five weeks of our first meeting, Carl was to be transferred to the oceanside city of Durban, eight hours' drive away.

In the meantime, after a few idyllic weeks, I was dying to hear from him the words "I love you." It may sound somehow infantile, but when you're in love these three words really mean something emotionally.

The time went all too fast, and suddenly it was Carl's last weekend in Johannesburg. We decided to spend it at Kyalami Ranch, a romantic resort hotel just outside the city.

It rained most of the weekend, but it made our togetherness more intense. Some of the most beautiful moments lovers can spend in bed are when the rain is splashing on the roof and beating against the windows. It was this way, just before dinner on Sunday night, that Carl declared his feelings.

"Xaviera," he started, cradling me in his arms, "I haven't told you how I felt before this because I wanted to be sure myself. I am not like some kid who makes rash statements to every woman he meets so he can get her into bed.

"The truth is that I love you."

I thought I would sail through the ceiling. I was like a teenager; I never felt those emotions before. Everything I ever wanted in my life was wrapped up in that moment in the cottage. For me this was the beginning of my life.

Then Carl went on: "And I would like to ask you whether you would consider becoming my wife."

Would I? If it had been up to me, I would have married him that day. That minute. But his idea was to spend more time together and get married after I came to the States and met his family.

In order that we would get to know each other better, Carl suggested I join him in Durban, where he was to stay for another two months, and just as soon as I could get free of my job and sublet my apartment, that's just what I did.

A few days before Christmas I joined Carl in Durban and moved into his airy apartment that we never did bother to furnish because we wouldn't be staying there very long. We never even had a gas stove, so we had all our meals in the best local restaurants.

Durban is a picturesque city with magnificent surfing beaches that are regarded as among the best in the world. I used to love going to them and watching the young, strong boys with their sun-bleached hair carrying surfboards under their arms. Dotted along the beaches were colorful kiosks belonging to the Indians selling hot dogs, pastries, and ice creams. Gypsy women would wander up and down selling their merchandise as well, which was usually dresses, sandals, or flowers.

The weather was hot and humid, and the strong sun streaming through the curtainless windows would wake us up, bathed in sweat, very early in the mornings. But it didn't bother us—we would make passionate love, then run across the road and jump into the ocean.

After Carl left for work each day I would shop for fruits and go back to the beach, where he would join me before lunch for a swim. He had been an Olympic swimmer in Rome, and I adored watching his powerful body plowing through the huge waves. Afterward we would stroll along the beach, and I believe people would consider us a happy, good-looking couple. Carl with his perpetual suntan and dark, curly hair and me a streaked blonde.

Nights we would spend dining, either alone or with some of his colleagues. Afterward we would always come home and make love again, for hours, chatting, laughing, eating fruit from each other's body. We were already becoming slaves to each another. Carl was a very strong man and could climax five times in two hours, and he had become a perfect lover.

Time was floating deliciously by. No fights, no hassles, and I was sure this was ultimate happiness. I didn't even *look* at another man apart from the surfers. All I cared for was Carl, my lover, my life.

After leaving Durban, we spent a two-month vacation roaming footloose and fancy free all over the east part of Africa, and this glorious countryside must be among some of the most spectacular on the face of the earth.

We saw Kruger National Park, with its zebras, wildebeests, elephants, lions, beautiful deer, and I was almost molested by a rhinoceros.

The last stop on our photo safari was Mozambique, where the weather was so hot that even the swimming pool at the hotel was too warm to be refreshing. It was there that we parted company temporarily.

Carl set out for America, and I went back to South Africa to tie up loose ends and earn enough money to pay my fare to the U.S. with Carl, the American citizen, sponsoring my visa.

On the way back to the States, Carl made a detour through Amsterdam to meet my parents and officially ask for my hand in marriage. My father had already been the victim of a massive stroke that left him paralyzed and without the power of speech, but my mother was very impressed by Carl's gallant behavior and was so proud I had chosen such a fine man.

For the next six months we exchanged letters of such sizzling passion that I am surprised the pages didn't ignite. And, two months before I was to leave for America, I returned to Holland to spend the last of my single days with my family.

Amsterdam in the rain—what a contrast from sun-soaked South Africa! My mother was waiting for me at the airport, and I noticed how she had aged. My father had suffered a second stroke, and the following day I went to see him in the hospital.

I was shocked at the sight of him, lying inert in the darkened room. He seemed to have shriveled, and there were deep hollows around his eyes. He gazed at me without speaking, but with a strangely furtive look. Something was wrong. I looked around and noticed that his little traveling clock was missing. He took that clock everywhere. I remembered its thick glass front, and a ghastly suspicion flashed through my mind. I pulled away the sheet, which was tucked unnaturally right up to his chin, and revealed the dried blood and the gashes on his wrist and throat. He had been physically too weak to sever the arteries with the slivers of glass from the clock, and his great, sad eyes seemed to implore me to finish what he had attempted. To whisper to me required all the strength he could muster.

"My child, you cannot know how much I have missed you. And now when at last you come home, you find me like this, a pitiful wreck, a burden on your mother. And if I linger on, I shall bring you and her nothing but sorrow. If you love me, pray for me to die."

He went on talking, but his sentences grew less coherent, as he succumbed to waves of weakness. I could not bring myself to tell him that he would soon be better; he was a doctor and would have seen my assurances as mere wishful thinking which deceived neither him nor me. I tried to fight back my tears— tears for his despair and his hopeless condition, tears for my mother and her lonely suffering, and tears of remorse that I had flown away and enjoyed myself when I should have been by her side. How selfish I had been in contrast to her uncomplaining, devoted self-sacrifice!

Back home I was still shaken, and I wandered the streets feverishly, hoping to see some friendly face, but my mind was on getting away to join Carl, the man I loved.

I was to leave for America in August, but a week before departure I got a long-distance call from Carl in Jamaica asking me could I possibly delay my trip.

"Something has developed that necessitates my staying here," he faltered. And even on the blurry transatlantic wire, I suspected from his tone that the development was not exactly office business.

That night I sat down and wrote him a long letter telling him what I feared, and asking him to let me know if he had met another woman. "I'm not so narrow-minded I would expect a virile man like you to lead a monastic life, but don't fall in love with someone else," I implored.

Carl's long, loving reply to that letter was reassuring.

"I promise you, Xaviera, you are the only woman I want in my life, and I am looking forward to being with you for the rest of our lives from next December to forever."

Four

Dutch Treat

*N*ew York's bustling Kennedy Airport on that December 1967 morning felt like the most uncharitable place on earth. Stampeding crowds jostled me, and Carl was nowhere in sight. Six o'clock was an uncivilized hour to arrive in the New World, but when you can afford only a cheap charter flight, you have no choice.

Despair was starting to consume me as the customs inspector chalked my last piece of luggage, when at last Carl's familiar face came into view. I spotted him first, ran over, and threw my arms around his neck ready for a kiss, but he turned his face away.

Was kissing your fiancé in a public airport anything to be embarrassed about? What the hell was going on?

"I'll get a skycap to carry your bags" were his only words as he led me from the arrival hall toward his huge American car.

"Welcome to the USA," he said as we crossed to the parking

area. Boy, some welcome! I had no gloves on, my coat was inadequate against the biting winds, and here the man who for the last eight months had sent me passionate letters, cards, and cables was behaving like a stranger.

Something, other than his conservative hairstyle and absent suntan, was different about him, and I had to know what it was. "Carl, is there something I should know about?" I asked. He switched on the car radio and answered with an awkward cough.

"Carl, I have given up everything I had to come here and be with you," I said. "So, if something has come between us, I believe I have a right to know."

Somehow I sensed if he told me anything it would be a lie, but I would settle for a half-truth. "Have you met another woman?"

He shifted uncomfortably on his side of the seat. "There *was* another woman," he began clumsily, "a legal secretary I met at an economists conference in Jamaica earlier this year." Her name was Rona, he said. The woman, according to Carl, was the mother of an eight-year-old son, in her mid-thirties, and crazy about him. However, he did not return her feelings and had slept with her maybe three times, no more, guaranteed.

"Okay, now I feel better," I said, and changed the subject.

We arrived at Carl's penthouse in the East Seventies to refresh and rest. The apartment was impressive, full of French provincial furniture and expensive antiques, but nothing interfered with the orderliness, not even one little flower with a note to say welcome home. It looked as though the decorator had departed only five minutes before.

We dropped the bags inside and went up to a tavern in Germantown for a quick bite to eat and then back home to take a bath, unpack, and make love—and something certainly was different.

Carl's strange attitude was contagious, and he did not turn me on at all; in fact, his big cock hurt me. We put on our bathrobes and turned on the television.

Around ten that night we felt more at ease with each other and started our lovemaking all over again. This time the old feelings were creeping back when the phone rang. Carl pulled away from me abruptly and picked it up.

And I kid you not—that next twenty-minute conversation certainly sounded as though he would rather be making love with whoever was on the other end than with me.

I was too deflated to ask any questions, and just rolled over and tried to sleep.

The next day was Sunday, and I thought Carl would show me the city, but around lunchtime he told me: "Xaviera, I have to go see my mother and give her a hand with an art exhibition she is helping open today. So please forgive me for leaving you alone for a while. Watch TV or write your folks a letter, and when I come back around six, we'll go out for a nice dinner."

Alone in the apartment I was confused and miserable. After all those months, couldn't he make himself available to take his fiancée somewhere on her first whole day in America?

The afternoon dragged by; six o'clock came and went, then seven, eight, nine, ten—and still no Carl. There was no food in the fridge, and I was very hungry and feeling sorry for myself. By ten-fifteen, when Carl returned, I was lying on the bed in tears.

Next morning he left early for work, and again by ten that night he had not returned home. When the phone rang, I answered it on the chance that it might be him.

"Who is this?" a strangely accented woman's voice demanded.

"My name is Xaviera, Carl Gordon's fiancée," I answered. "And who is this?"

There was a stunned silence, then her reply: "My name is Rona Wong—and Carl Gordon is *my* fiancé."

The voice started relating a story, some of which I already knew, of how, where, and why they had met.

"Tell me," I asked. "How come you're in New York?"

"Carl asked me to come here from Kingston and marry him." Rona told me of Carl's urging, and under his sponsorship she had tossed up her job, left her son with friends, and come to New York five months before.

However, since arriving all she'd had from Carl were promises, promises, and more of the same.

"Carl keeps postponing the wedding date, and I have no money, and being an alien, I am not allowed to work," she said, and started to cry.

Distressed though I was at her call, I felt kind of sorry for her—and also a little curious as to what my rival looked like—so I agreed to come down to her place.

The address she gave was Sutton Place, not far from where his parents lived, and if hearing her story surprised me, seeing the woman at her door really amazed me.

Carl had been something of a racist in South Africa, yet this woman I was now confronting—who claimed to be his fiancée—was a black Oriental!

Not only that, she had protruding teeth, dumpy legs, and bushy, kinky hair. Some kind of competition I had.

Inside I admired a potted poinsettia plant. "Thank you," she said. "Carl gave it to me yesterday."

So this was the "mother" he had to neglect his fiancée to see? The more I heard, the more urgent it seemed to demand an explanation from Carl. So Rona and I decided to phone and ask him over.

Carl answered the phone when I called the house and said he'd been worrying about where I could be.

"I'm in the Sutton Place area," I said. "But not at your parents' home." And he guessed right away where I was. There was nothing he could do but come down there and face the music.

While we were waiting for Carl, Rona gave me a cup of China tea and some delicious homemade cookies. She was a homey person and described proudly the exotic meals which she cooked for Carl. But the moment he walked through the door, she started to yell at him at the top of her voice.

"You cheating bastard! Make up your fucking mind. Which of us do you want to marry?"

"All that crap about visiting your mother!" I chimed in. "You were off to see *her,* weren't you?"

"What mother?" interrupted Rona. "You know that dumb jerk was too ashamed to introduce me to his mother, just because I am black. So, one day I took myself off on my own to meet his folks."

"What happened?" I asked. It was as though Carl no longer existed.

"That alcoholic bitch! She treated me like shit. She pretended to think that I was applying for a job as a maid and told me that as they already had a Japanese girl, a Jamaican would make a nice color scheme." She turned back to Carl. "Well?" she demanded.

"Well," Carl stammered, "Xaviera is my official fiancée because I have been to Holland and got her father's consent. As a matter of fact," he continued, "she did actually move in with me a few days ago."

That was enough for Rona. In a fury, she grabbed a heavy stone ashtray and aimed it at Carl's head.

Luckily, I was close enough to prevent her from throwing it, but in that critical moment I thought I saw something that I hoped I had mistaken. As my fiancé was threatened with danger, a look of erotic pleasure flashed in his eyes!

The moment quickly passed, and we left. I felt sorry for Rona, but I was very much in love with Carl and so glad he had chosen me in her presence that I accepted his mumbled explanation and agreed not to bring up the matter again. I can easily forgive when I'm in love. And what else could I do? I knew no one else in New York. I was also broke and didn't have the fare to go back home.

Two days after that Sutton Place drama, I was in for another interesting introduction into Carl's intimate life—his family.

Carl's parents were both doctors and owned a beautiful duplex cooperative apartment. The inside of the apartment was truly magnificent, and huge enough to have both a Japanese and a Greek maid to run it.

Carl's father, a charming, gentle introvert, had been house physician to the Kennedys at the White House. His mother was very different. A dermatologist, she made me itch to be a long way away from her. She was small, wiry, and very plain, and would spend the whole day gossiping in a harsh, strident voice which had been coarsened by incessant smoking and soaking—in gin!

She confirmed a most unfavorable impression, which I had by then formed of wealthy New York women. The older they were, the sillier and more juvenile were their clothes, and all their layers of makeup, rows of false eyelashes, and uniform Vidal Sassoon hairdos simply made them look even more ridiculous, as they paraded around Bloomingdale's or Bonwit Teller's counters. Growing old was apparently a sin. Was it a sense of insecurity or a lack of love which compelled these caricature-women to try to compete with their own daughters? Carl's mother was one of these "eternally young."

Carl himself was a real mama's boy, but his younger brother, Jimmy, a sweet, quiet young man of twenty-four, was very like his father, serious, hardworking, and critical. The fifth member of the Gordon household was Dudley, a tiny, toothless Yorkshire terrier, which Mrs. Gordon fussed over and pampered, as well she might, for he was the only one of the family who listened to her nonsense. She and the dog used to wear identical ribbons; I judged that the dog was the better-looking partner.

From our first introduction, I don't think that woman cared for me. I tried to be natural and spontaneous with her, and she was insecure and phony with me. And, to be candid, I didn't endear myself when I replied to her bad French the way the language is spoken in France.

However, I had to try to get along with the Gordons because I was going to be their daughter-in-law if, indeed, the day ever came.

It was three months after I arrived in America, and I was still not married. I was living with Carl, and my visa was expiring. I pointed out that if we weren't married soon I would have to leave the country, but this didn't hurry him up. "Get a job at a consulate and get a diplomatic visa," he said.

So I took a job in a foreign consulate, and just as well, because I started needing money.

Soon after I arrived here I learned that the free-spending Carl in South Africa was a man very much on an expense account. In New York there were no lavish meals or any presents. Carl was even so stingy that he wouldn't pay my dry-cleaning bill. He paid the food and the rent, but everything else was at my expense. He even got mad at me one time when he saw me sending money home to my family.

"Carl, I have been educated by my parents in a good way," I reminded him. "I studied music, speak five languages, and have traveled all over Europe with them. They have given me the best they could, so why should I neglect them now after my father's long illness had left him in bad financial shape?" And I sent them something from my salary every month.

Another thing I was disturbed to find out about Carl was his anti-Semitism. I knew his mother had changed her religion to Presbyterian, and Carl, it seemed, also did everything he could to conceal his Jewish origins. The family had even changed its Jewish surname.

Carl was a member of the supposedly anti-Semitic New York Athletic Club, and once, when he took me there for a fencing competition, he made me conceal my Star of David pendant. "Hide it in your sweater," he whispered, "and they'll never know you're Jewish, because you don't look it."

Other times, when people were coming for dinner, he would make me hide the thing I treasured most, a valuable copper menorah, which was a gift from my family, and the only possession of sentimental worth I had in this country.

The last thing he did before guests arrived was to check if the menorah was out of sight. "Put that candle in a drawer," he would say, which to me was like burying your pride.

After six months in America the subject of marriage was being discussed less and less, and at this point I didn't dare mention it for fear he would yell at me.

In spring I remember walking through Central Park, seeing the pregnant women or the married couples with their children, and feeling jealous of them because they were living legitimately with their husbands and could raise a family the way it should be. And what was I doing? Living as Carl's common-law wife.

I would have loved to have a baby with Carl. I was sure it would be beautiful. I wanted a boy first, then a girl. Some nights in the heat of passion, Carl would even say, "Darling, don't use your diaphragm tonight, I want to make you a baby."

I wouldn't obey him, because, as much as I wanted it, I did not want a baby without being married. And I would not use that as a weapon to get him to marry me, because whenever I mentioned marriage these days he would lash out at me and say, "Don't push it." Also, at that time I found out something I never knew before—that he had just got officially divorced from his first wife. No wonder he didn't want to marry me in South Africa: he would have been a bigamist!

Carl's passionate words were just words—empty of any real meaning—I found out one time when I was three weeks late with my period. I had not yet seen a doctor, but I told Carl I was feeling nauseous.

He went into a rage and started screaming that he didn't want to be pushed into anything, and insisted on an abortion. That was the last thing I would do. I would never kill something inside me that was going to be a human being, especially when the father was the one and only man I loved and was supposed to be marrying.

Carl kept yelling words so humiliating and ugly that I slipped away into the bathroom and swallowed a handful of sleeping pills.

When I came back into the room, Carl was still being wildly abusive. A wave of faintness swept over me. My limbs grew numb, and my whole body went limp. Suddenly, I could no longer bear his harsh language, and there seemed no point in living. In a daze, I stumbled out onto the balcony and, teetering on the rail, I gazed down at the myriad twinkling lights of Manhattan beckoning me, while Carl's voice droned on monotonously in the background. To let go was a temptation, to be rid of his accusations and lies, and of a hysterical mother-in-law.

Carl must have realized what was going through my mind, for his recriminations gave way to entreaties.

"Xaviera, don't do it!" he cried. "Think what the neighbors would say. I really do love you, and we don't want a scandal, do we?"

It was his genteel hypocrisy which nauseated me. Why the hell should I take my life for the sake of such a disgusting phony? I remembered the love which my mother had lavished on me and my father's steadfast courage. Suicide would be a betrayal of them and all that they had sacrificed for me. So I let Carl guide me back into the room.

I woke up after it was dark the next day, and Carl was there with red roses and gentle words, trying to be the old Carl.

In an effort to compensate, he suggested we spend a long weekend with his parents at their big house in the Hamptons. If he'd said let's spend a weekend in the Women's House of Detention, it couldn't have been less appealing to me. But I went along with any effort he made to keep our engagement alive, even though by this time the thought of his mother made me choke, and I was sure the feelings were mutual.

The weekend came around, and his mother outdid herself in meanness. Even though she was aware we had now lived together for more than half a year, and there was no reason to "keep up appearances," she pointedly assigned me a bedroom on one floor and Carl a room at the other side of the house on a different floor. She even went as far as locking the freaky little dog in Carl's room at night so that if I came in or he went out, the toothless little beast would bark. And she was not satisfied to stop there. This woman, who had lived in Manhattan all her life, went into his room at two in the morning to ask him the New York telephone code.

Carl's mother was so possessive about her son that if there were a law allowing her to marry him, she would have done so. He also had a mother complex, but not based on sentiment. She once threatened to disinherit him if he married me, and the thought of missing out on her money almost gave him a coronary.

The weekend was, as expected, thoroughly depressing, and I spent most of the time staying out of the way to avoid a scene. Her husband had not come along, preferring to go fishing and— I suspect—keep as far as possible from his wife's insane babble. So I spent most of my time at the piano because I had studied the classics for twelve years, and it always gives me great pleasure to play. And at least it gave me something to do.

When the last afternoon mercifully arrived, I was sitting, reading a book, in the room off the entrance hall when Mrs. Gordon came out to answer a ring at the doorbell.

From where I was sitting I could see that outside was a gorgeous seventeen-year-old boy with a suntan and shoulder-length blond hair.

Her hatchet expression immediately changed to her version of a smile. "Hi," she croaked. "What can I do for you?"

"Is this Dr. Johnson's house?" the beautiful boy said.

"Why, no, I'm Dr. Goldman." She always preferred to be called by her professional name. "Will I do?"

"I'm looking for Dr. Johnson," the boy said impatiently. "Isn't this his house?"

"No, it's not, but come in anyway and let me pour you a drink." She giggled grotesquely.

"No, thank you, ma'am, this is an emergency," he said, and hurried away.

Mrs. Gordon shut the door, smiled at herself in the hall mirror, and adjusted her bow, and for the first time noticed me sitting there.

"Why, Xaviera," she said, blushing and flushing, "you're there!" Then she added: "Did you see that? What was it, a boy or a girl?"

"If that was a girl," I said, "you would not have been jumping up and down like some jack-in-the-box. You were like Blanche in *A Streetcar Named Desire*—trying to seduce a seventeen-year-old boy." At that moment the phone rang, and she answered it and was grateful for the interruption. But I had already said too much, and I knew the old harridan would not rest until she had my scalp on her belt. In the car on the way back to New York she went after it.

As usual, Mrs. Gordon was sitting up front beside her darling son, Carl, and I, the fiancée, was banished by myself in the back. Her incessant chatter got onto the subject of housing in general, and, at her engineering, in Holland in particular.

"I guess the rentals for apartments must be very high in Amsterdam," she said.

"Oh, why?"

"Because it seems to me Dutch girls have the habit of moving in with their boyfriends without marrying them, and there has to be a reason."

To me, this was the last drop in the bucket. I couldn't keep quiet anymore.

"Mrs. Gordon," I began, "it is not from choice that I live in an unmarried state with your son . . . If you can stretch your little brain under that bleached hair and recall, your son officially proposed to me through my parents, brought me here on a false promise of marriage, and set me up in his home on a temporary arrangement, which has now been going on for nine months.

"What's more, I paid my own fare, and I am now working to support myself in order to get a place of my own. So altogether the Dutch treat has been on me!"

But I didn't stop there. All my pent-up anger had to be released on this dreadful woman.

"I have put up with a lot of nonsense from you, too. Your trite phone calls in the middle of the night. Your home is as warm and welcoming as a funeral parlor. If your maid is out, you are too idle even to give somebody a drink. And when I do go to the fridge, even the tonic bottle is filled with gin."

"What are you saying?" Carl interrupted my tirade. "Gin? In a tonic bottle?"

"Just that. Your mother is a secret boozer. Your father has been trying to cut down her drinking, so she has taken to stashing the stuff away in tonic or soda bottles. No wonder that your husband has not slept with you for ten years," I snapped at Mrs. Gordon.

"What?" she shrieked in a fury. "Who told you that?"

"Your own dear son, Carl," I replied.

Carl would have liked a great hole to open in the floor of his car and swallow him up, but I had not finished with his mother.

"You have the nerve to criticize my family. May I remind you that my father was a respected physician, a Jew who lost everything in the war when all of my family was imprisoned in concentration camps, while you sat back and read about that sort of thing in your newspapers. But he was not so spineless as to change his name and his religion. As for you, Mrs. Gordon, you would not be so contemptible a creature if you stopped trying to look like a teenager, and acted with a bit more dignity and graciousness."

With that she whirled around and slapped me hard across the face.

Carl never said a word during the whole tirade, nor did he speak now, even though I had hoped he would come to my defense. And the rest of the trip was spent in agonized silence.

I knew that Mrs. Gordon would be determined, however, to have a final word, and as we dropped her off on Sutton Place, she hissed, "I'll see you on a plane back to Holland. I'll get you deported. Who are you, anyway? You're nothing, not even an immigrant." She stalked into the house and slammed the door.

Back at our apartment, as Carl and I undressed to take a shower, nothing had been said, because I was waiting for him to break the silence with an apology to me.

Instead he started yelling: "Don't you ever address my mother like that again!" he raged. "Now you have absolutely wrecked all our marriage plans." As if he had any intention anyway.

Then he grabbed a wooden coat hanger and raised it to hit me. A man striking a woman is the last thing I can stand. It's cowardly and animalistic.

"How dare your mother hit me with her hand!" I screamed back. "And how dare you threaten to hit me now, bastard!" I was so furious that if I had had a knife I would have stabbed him. But the closest weapon was a heavy antique clothes brush his grandfather had bequeathed him, and I grabbed it and started thrashing him wildly. I also used my nails to tear at his flesh, and he was getting black and blue and bleeding when all of a sudden I saw in his eyes the same weird erotic look he had the night Rona threatened to kill him.

I glanced down, and he'd got this huge erection. By now I was all confused, but the erotic moment quickly passed, and we got into a real fistfight, which, for us, was the beginning of the end.

From that lousy Sunday we took turns sleeping on the living-room sofa until I found a place to share with another Dutch girl named Sonia, who worked on my floor at Rockefeller Plaza, at the Dutch consulate.

Her apartment was only a few blocks from Carl's, and I still kept most of my things there and stayed with him several nights a week.

But moving out, I thought, was the only way I might ingratiate myself slightly with his parents and redeem our turbulent romance. It sounds crazy, but I still loved the man despite everything, and we were still slaves to each other's bodies.

Carl went away frequently on trips during that period, and there were times I would be so hurt and lonely I would have to soothe my bruised emotions with some gay girl I met in a bar around the corner called the Tree.

When the Olympic Games were held in Mexico City in October 1968, Carl announced that he was going to take a vacation by himself and go there. This time he went away for longer than usual. Before he left I vaguely recall casually mentioning that I had a light-skinned Indonesian girlfriend named Penny, who was going to attend the Olympic Games as a representative for our national airline, KLM. I thought nothing about it at the time.

I was very depressed while he was gone, and I had a longer than usual affair with a girl from the Dominican Republic whom I picked up at the gay bar. Even though it was only a woman I cheated with, I told Carl about it when he returned, and his pride was hurt. And, what is almost laughable, he said after that admission marriage would be impossible because he would never be able to trust his wife while he was away on a business trip.

What a hypocrite. I was sure he was doing something more in Mexico City for a month than just watching the hundred-meter dash. But I had no proof of anything, at least not at the time. In spite of his attitude, I couldn't leave him. Love is blind! Stupid, also, when it blinds one to a mate's cruelty.

Around the time Carl came back from Mexico City, a strange change was occurring in his lovemaking, and he was becoming slightly freaky.

One night while we were making love, he said to me, "Why don't you pick up that antique clothes brush and just beat me up a little?"

That was just kid stuff compared to what he wanted later on. He would ask me to talk dirty about the girls I made it with and how I would suck their pussies and their tits. He also liked me to dress up in slinky clothes and do a striptease for him while he lay around in his bathrobe with the front open. He wanted me to brush against his arm with my sleeve or my scarf and jump away to tease him.

As he became kinkier, I went out and bought some sex-perversion books to learn new things to please him. I taught myself the Japanese trick of inserting a string of pearls in his back passage and removing them one at a time to excite him, and all at once to make him climax.

Then he started saying, "Xaviera, I want to be your whore. Make me your whore." So I bought a dildo through a lesbian friend, and I would insert it, sit on his back like a jockey, with a riding crop in my hand, and pretend I was riding him at Aqueduct. I would call the race as I whipped him along to the finish line, and each time, of course, I had to announce that he was the winner. I also remember giving seductive striptease performances while he lay on the couch, teasing him and teasing him and finally raping him.

Toward the end, the last thing he wanted was straight sex anymore, and I wondered where on earth this sick situation was going to end.

Soon after, Carl came up with the answer. One day he told me he was being transferred to São Paulo, Brazil.

"Don't get upset, Xaviera," he said. "This separation could be the best thing for us." He was to leave in the middle of February, and suggested I plan to join him around May, and definitely we would be married. He promised.

The actual day he left was Valentine's Day, and for a few days before that he became very secretive and would not let me clear out the mailbox. Valentine's Day does not mean much to me, but I started to suspect it meant something more to him.

There's something he's hiding, I thought, but I couldn't figure out what. The night before his departure, we stayed together, and the next morning while he was taking one of those long baths in all the bubbles that he liked, I decided to find out.

I had an idea that the clue to our relationship now and in the future was inside his black attaché case, which he always kept locked and which was now lying on the sofa. The last thing I like to be is a snoop, but this action was justified because I could feel he was holding something very important from me.

Knowing the way Carl's mind worked, I figured out that the combination to the attaché case had to be something obvious. I tried 353, 747, 636, 545, and was getting very nervous that he might come out and catch me. So I peeped in the door, and there he was lying in his bubbles and reading his paper.

The fourteenth combination, 242, opened it, and inside I found five Valentine cards from five different senders, and one registered letter. The letter was in a familiar handwriting, and the stamp was from Holland. My hands were shaking as I opened it.

"My dearest Mexican Globo," it began. "I hope this letter gets into your hands safely, because I would hate Xaviera to read it, since we are still good friends. I can't tell you how happy I am, and our Mexican love affair is still freshly printed on my mind. My darling, I am all excited. Your beautiful marriage proposal is the most fabulous present I have ever had. I am dying to depart from Holland. I could not think of a nicer person to spend the rest of my life with. I am jealous of Xaviera for every moment she has spent with you lately, and I count the days until we meet. See you in Sâo Paulo. Your Indonesian Penny."

Five

What's a Girl Like Me?

By that bleak February day in 1969 when Carl left for Brazil, my confidence in myself as a woman and a human being was at an all-time low.

I was battle scarred from two whole years of being in love with and faithful to a man who cheated, humiliated, and finally abandoned me. And for the first time in my reasonably well-adjusted life, I had an inferiority complex you could photograph.

I desperately needed warmth and reassurance, and an obvious easy way was to hear men praise me as a lover. I had thrown Carl out of my house after showing him the letter from Indonesian Penny. He called several times to apologize, but I hung up on him. His plane was to take off at four that same afternoon, and by that time I was in bed screwing my brains out with a man I'd met at Maxwell's Plum.

This was the first man I had been with since I first met my fiancé, and to tell you the truth, it was a dismal failure. We were both looking for something neither of us got. The baby-faced lawyer wanted a no-strings, uncomplicated roll in the feathers, and I wanted an escape from my misery. But instead of feeling elated with his loving, I burst into tears and sent him away.

Nevertheless, I decided my stolen self-esteem was in a bed somewhere in Manhattan, so for the next six months I cut a sexual swath a mile wide across the city.

After work each day I would go to the bars where the gray-flannel set hung out, like Ratazzi, P. J. Clarke's, Ad Lib, Charley-O's, or Maxwell's Plum. Charley-O's was downstairs in my building, and the junior-executive types would go there to get laid before the last train to Westport.

These men would all be full of promises about how they could introduce you to this job, or get you cut-rate travel or whatever it was they thought you might want. Meanwhile, you'd end up in bed with them, and when you'd call the next day they were always out.

My roommate, Sonia, who knew me from the suffering days when I was living with Carl, took a genuine big-sisterly interest in me, but sometimes she would get angry enough to call me a nymphomaniac.

She was nine years older than me, unmarried, and disillusioned with life; her retreat from reality was the bottle, in the same way mine was sex. At night she would quietly drink herself into her happier world while I would screw myself into mine.

I would cruise the First Avenue singles bars where Brooklyn, Bronx, and Queens secretaries go looking for marriage and end up settling for a night in bed. My scene was to drag home any Tom, Harry, or Dick who had a pleasant face and a tolerable manner.

I went on that way until around August, when things got so depressingly repetitive and aimless I thought I would go around the bend. As providence had it, one of the junior execs actually came through with a round-trip ticket to Miami.

It was just the break I was waiting for, and although I knew nobody there, the change of scene would help my discontent.

The long weekend was spent swimming, sunbathing, and mixing in with a happy crowd of people from Miami. I even met a nice hillbilly who was the manager of an advertising agency. Vernon, from nearby Dinner Key, owned a luxurious yacht, and he soon had me as a housemate on his boat. We took trips with some of his young friends and had orgies almost every day. It was fun to go topless and shock the passing captains with their families. By Sunday night I was a much calmer, happier girl than the one who had arrived there the previous Wednesday evening.

There was only one small moment of drama in the whole trip, and that was when I was leaving. Somehow the airline had mixed up the tickets, and for a while it was uncertain whether I would be able to have my scheduled seat.

For some reason the ticket clerk was giving me a hard time, and I guessed it was because the man who was double-booked was much more influential than I. He sure looked it; he was an expensively dressed, distinguished-looking Englishman.

For ten minutes I argued furiously that I had to be back in time for work the next day, and finally won a place. However, I was surprised to see the tall Englishman—when we got off the plane at LaGuardia—walking purposefully toward me.

"Hi." He smiled. "My name is Evelyn St. John; I am English, and I live in Paris, and I'm here in New York for a week." A mouthful for openers.

"I am also ashamed of myself for hoping you would get bumped off the flight because I was after your seat," he continued. "So by way of apology, would you let me take you out on the town tonight?"

I felt immediately attracted to him. He was charming, and handsome, with prematurely gray hair.

"It's about midnight now," I said, "so what can we do?"

"Let's start off with a drink at my hotel and take it from there."

In the taxi on the way to the Hilton, Evelyn said, "Why not check in with me tonight? Are you married or single?"

"No, I'm not married, I live with a square roommate. I like you and have nothing to lose." As has been established, I daresay, I was never very inhibited about sex.

That night I moved in with him, and he became the first man I felt anything for in the six months since Carl had left me. We made love all through the night, and in the morning I went straight from his bed to my office, without a wink of sleep.

Love can elate you in a way that a month of early nights never can, and I confess I thought I was in love.

Evelyn was what I could only describe as a truly elegant lover. Considerate, controlled, yet very passionate. You could tell he had penetrated the best beds in Europe in the arms of the most sophisticated women.

Not that he consciously let it be known. Quite the contrary. He had the most convincing way of breathing undying love when he was on that paradise stroke. He was that perfect combination men expect only in a woman: a cultivated lady in the living room and an animal maniac in bed.

Evelyn was witty, urbane, generous—everything Carl and the others were not.

For the next week I spent the days dreaming about the nights. After work each day I would float across the half block between my office and the Hilton to meet my lover for romantic dinners, concerts, Broadway shows, and passion. It was a fantastic relationship, sexual and cerebral, and no wonder I was in love—or thought I was—and showed it in every way.

But Evelyn had another way of demonstrating his feeling for me. A way I have since learned is typical of people of his breeding and background, and, to my horror, he exposed me to it toward the end of the week after a romantic dawn.

I remember vividly the setting for the conversation that was to change the entire course of my straight and simple life. He was leaning back against the pillow, and I was cradled in his arms.

"Xaviera," he began in his slow, Oxford-accented English. "I can never tell you in words just how wonderful you have made this week in New York."

I shuddered at the reminder that today was Friday, and on Sunday he would leave. "To show you what you have meant, I have something for you," he went on.

"What is it?" I asked dreamily. I was always on a cloud after we made love.

"Here," he said, and handed me a hundred-dollar bill.

I froze. I was shocked, hurt, and speechless with anger. At least if this was not love on his part, he had no right to make it seem like prostitution.

My mother had always told me not to accept money from any man except the man I marry. "If a man friend insists on giving you something, ask for flowers or chocolates" was her advice.

"Evelyn," I said when the numbness wore off, "you make me feel like a whore. I don't want your hundred dollars; here it is, please take it back."

He was genuinely surprised, but he persisted.

"I know your father is ill, Xaviera, so take the money and send it to your mother so that she can buy a present for him."

He took an envelope from the drawer, told me to address it to my mother, and put the money inside. Then he got dressed, and went out to mail it. That made me feel better, because I did not use the money myself.

Next day Evelyn took me to Saks and bought me $800 worth of dresses, shoes, and handbags, and whatever else I wanted. And this, to me, was the really tremendous gesture of a gentleman, and he was the first man who ever bought me anything of value.

During my engagement to Carl, I was the one who spent half my salary to give him a birthday or Christmas present, or, when I could not afford it, spent hours writing poems for him. He gave me nothing in return, except his insincere promises.

So Evelyn had truly impressed me with his behavior, and he gave me some advice before he left for Paris the next day.

"A girl like you should let men spoil her," he said. "You are worth a lot more than a dinner here and a show there. You should be kept and cared for financially.

"You have all the qualities a man should pay for. You're attractive, intelligent, good company, happy, gay, and on top of everything, you genuinely love sex."

Previously I had met girls who had sugar-daddy types in the background, but I was always too proud to ask anyone for anything. I was not "mistress material." And, even though I had been shocked when Evelyn St. John gave me the money, after he treated me so nicely it occurred to me that it wouldn't be so bad to have this happen more often.

It would have been wonderful if Evelyn had asked me to return to Paris with him, but of course I understood why he could not. He was, after all, a married man.

But after he left, I went back to happily screwing my brains out all over town and having men take advantage of my constant horniness.

My job at the consulate was really boring me now, too, because it was routine and unchallenging.

The rare bright moments were when I met some nice man who called in for legal or some other kind of advice. One of them, a Dutchman named Dirk, called up one day to have his passport renewed.

As we got turned on to each other's voices on the phone, I got the impression he was very handsome because he certainly sounded it, and after talking for about ten minutes he said, "Forget about business—why don't we meet today for lunch?"

I met Dirk at a restaurant across from Rockefeller Center, and while he was not exactly as handsome as he somehow sounded, he was a charming, spontaneous kind of man.

At lunch we talked about his private life and his twenty-year-old marriage that now existed only in name and how he just lived for his job and his children.

I asked him bluntly what he did about his sex life. Did he have a girlfriend?

"No, I just use call girls when I need them," he said. At that time, to show you how innocent I was in some areas, I did not exactly know what call girls were.

I knew they were not listed in the yellow pages, but I thought it was a service you called if you wanted a black girl with big tits or a Chinese girl with no tits, on a rental basis and not for a one-shot session. More like an employment agency.

Dirk was a man in his mid-forties, so I supposed men at that time of life did that kind of thing.

When lunch was over, he suggested we meet after work to go somewhere and be alone. I willingly agreed. After all, I had made it with half of Rockefeller Center, so why deny my own countryman?

It so happened that Sonia was away on three weeks' leave, so I suggested my place at 6:00 P.M. He was eager, and I was looking forward to some exciting sex with a man who was a nice, humorous person.

But things weren't to be exactly as I expected. It turned out that Dirk was utterly impotent and got his kicks freaking out on the phone with other girls in between performing cunnilingus on me.

After an hour he had to leave, but I could tell he had had a good time, and even though he was no Valentino, I enjoyed his company also.

And recent history repeated itself that night. After he got dressed, Dirk took out his wallet and handed me $150.

I was dumbfounded, but not for the same reason as with Evelyn St. John. The amount was what astounded me. Evelyn gave me $100 for a whole week of making love, and Dirk gave me more for an hour of not making it!

He also gave me a lecture similar to Evelyn's, but something even more constructive.

"Xaviera, if you are going to make money out of this, we have to help you meet the right people. And you should. Why give all that pleasure away?"

By this time I was in complete agreement. "Okay," I said, "let's do something about it."

Dirk dialed a number, and a raucous female voice picked up on the other end. "Who is it?" she yelled.

"It's Dirk here, Pearl, and I have someone I think you ought to meet." Pearl Greenberg was a small-time madam, and Dirk was a sometime client of hers.

He told her all about me and recommended we get together for the benefit of us both.

"Sure," she screamed into the phone in a happy voice. "Get her over here, and she can start work tonight."

Dirk gave me an address down on the wrong part of Ninth Street in Greenwich Village, where I had to be at eight o'clock. I had one problem, though—I didn't know what prostitutes wear to work. I didn't want to wear what my image of them dictated: wigs, heavy makeup, tight clothes, and black stockings. To hell with it, I thought. I may behave as a prostitute, but I'll be damned if I'll dress like one. So I went *pura natura* in the blouse and skirt I had on.

The cab dropped me off at a shabby brownstone, and I ascended five flights of dusty stairs and knocked on my first whorehouse door.

"Who is it?" Pearl's raspy voice came through the door.

"It's Xaviera, you were expecting me," I called back. After a long minute of rattling of chains and shuttling of locks, the door fell open to reveal a homely big-boned girl, naked except for an Afro wig, with pendulous breasts threatening her ample waistline.

"Pleased ta meetcha," Pearl said. *"Ontray voo."*

I entered this whorish place with red curtains, and ragged carpet, and very messy with scarves, wigs, shortie pajamas, and assorted lingerie all over the place, and a projector for dirty movies.

In the middle of the room, lying face up on a sheet, was a fat man naked as the proverbial jaybird. Pearl had obviously been working him up, because his equipment was pointing skyward like the Statue of Liberty.

"Okay, this is your first victim." My hostess gestured to him. "Go ahead, baby, and fuck him." So I took off my clothes and jumped on top and fucked my brains out. I really enjoyed it, because he turned out to be a nice person, and his cock was as hard as a cock should be.

I could see he enjoyed me, too, and Pearl was out of her mind with the excitement of discovery—as she told everyone in Manhattan on the phone in the next hour. "I've got this lovely *Yiddishe madel* from Amsterdam who loves sex and will do anything you want," she broadcast.

So that was the beginning of a pleasant if not too profitable relationship with Pearl. She was what we call a *mensch* in Yiddish—good-hearted, good-humored, spontaneous, and warm.

Pearl had a black pimp somewhere in the background who kept her more or less on the poverty line. Her clients were mostly men from the garment district—not the bosses, but the middle-management guys who paid only $25 or $50 tops. I remember times when I would service my clients in their workrooms after the staff had left for the day.

The men, in three or fours, would pull two racks of dresses around to make an L-shaped screen and put some other garments on the floor and make love to me one by one.

Facilities were never the best, and one of them would always bring a roll of toilet paper to use in lieu of towels or showers. After I stood up following one of those two-hour sessions, I would have imprinted on my back impressions of zippers, hooks and eyes, buttons, and any other trimmings in their current line.

Pearl's financial arrangement with me was 40–60, so for every $25 date, I got $15. It wasn't much, but in quantity it did make a difference to my $150 from the consulate job.

For the first three weeks, I was able to take customers back to the apartment while Sonia was still out of town, but when she returned things became tough. I had to take them either to

Pearl's whory whorehouse all the way downtown, or borrow a crummy room belonging to a gay friend—and buy him a shirt or a bottle of aftershave as payment now and again.

Obviously that was not a satisfactory arrangement, and I still remember standing in the street weary and cold at 3:00 A.M. trying to get a taxi after a grueling night's work.

I had already solved the daytime transportation problem the way all Dutch people do, by buying a bicycle from my first earned money with Pearl. I would ride around to my lunchtime and early-evening assignments on this and save time and money.

When I first went into the business, I was extremely naive and not very discreet, probably because I saw no harm in what I was doing. From the beginning, I could justify to myself what the whole thing was about. However, the Saturday afternoon before Sonia came home, I was in for a nasty experience, because I had failed to cover my tracks. Two customers had just left, and while expecting another I was cleaning and oiling my bicycle when there was a ring at the doorbell. In my naïveté, I opened it without looking through the peephole, and a man in a blue uniform pushed his way in.

"I am an officer of the law," he announced. To me he looked more like a street fighter than a policeman. His uniform was crumpled, his nose was all over his face, and his front teeth were missing.

"Call me Mac, girlie," he said, and, uninvited, sat himself down. He opened his conversation with the accusation that I was a prostitute and there were complaints from several neighbors.

"Me, a prostitute?" I said. "All I am is a little secretary cleaning her bicycle and not bothering a soul. I work for a consulate, and you can check out my references."

"Why don't you pour me a Scotch on the rocks" was his

unpolicemanlike reply. This was my first brush with the law, and I was not thinking too straight, so I did as he requested.

In about five minutes I returned to the living room with his drink to find him marching around looking in closets, sorting out papers, and being generally very nosy.

Then he sat down again and started talking about nothing particularly connected with the law. Meanwhile, I had another customer due at any time, so I excused myself to go into the bedroom and change. But the fat policeman followed me.

All of a sudden I noticed his fly undone, and he was reaching inside to expose himself. Then he grabbed me and threw me screaming onto the bed. Even though he was supposed to be a policeman, my involuntary cry was "Help, police, help!"

He backed off, but started a verbal attack. "I want you to know, girlie, I live in Queens, and I have a wife and four kids, and my wife is pregnant again. And you girls make so much easy money, and I have to work like a dog for a lousy salary."

Innocent as I was, I knew what he was leading up to.

"I think you should start paying me a certain amount of money each week, and I will give you all the protection you want."

"No," I said, "I don't need protection, because I am doing nothing wrong."

"I'll tell you what, girlie," he said. "I'll leave, but think things over, and I'll be in touch."

Throughout the encounter, I kept my composure but was more frightened than I looked. After he went, I called up my next client, a psychiatrist, and told him about the incident.

"It seems like a phony-baloney deal to me," the shrink said. "They're trying to use scare tactics. Be more careful in the future, and in the meantime check your house to see if anything is missing."

After I hung up, I went inside to the bedroom, and the first thing my eyes fell on was the top of the bureau. Before the policeman arrived, it had contained $100, my day's income, and an expensive camera. Now it was bare.

Also missing, for some odd reason, was an envelope containing pornographic pictures Carl had taken of me alone and of us together. I chalked up the money and the camera to experience and was mad at my stupidity in leaving them around, but as for the pictures, I was soon to hear why they vanished.

When Sonia came back three days later, I told her what happened, leaving out the part about the customers, and she said I was very naive, because everyone knows a policeman has to show a search warrant. This last incident, however, put a further strain on our deteriorating relationship, and ruining my friendship with Sonia was the last thing I wanted to see happen.

Sonia was getting more suspicious every day. The phone never stopped ringing at all hours of the day and night, and almost all the calls were for me. The strain was destroying our friendship, so I resolved to tell her honestly and fully what was going on. The news certainly jolted her.

"Jesus!" she exclaimed. "You want to watch your step. For Christ's sake, be careful what types you bring home. As a foreigner, you could find yourself in a lot of trouble. And you can be sure that the Dutch consulate can't be kept in the dark forever. You don't have your green card, so if you lose the special status you enjoy from the consulate, you will have no right to work in this country, and you will not be able to stay legally.

"I must say, I don't know what attracts you to that sort of business. I could never sleep with a man for money; I really have to love a guy to sleep with him."

"You know for years Carl used to fuck me several times every day, and I got used to regular sex. It so happens that I like fucking." It was difficult to explain to Sonia how different our outlooks on life were. "The wives of my customers lead lives of luxury, yet they are always finding excuses for not letting their men have sex with them. So I was satisfying a need, and why not get paid for it? And as I have become more professional, I no longer feel merely used by men. They treat me with the respect due to a real businesswoman."

Sonia shook her head, and we came to the decision that it would be better if we stopped living together. She was lucky enough to find a charming rent-controlled apartment, and when she moved out, I stayed on and had no difficulty in affording the rent of $285 a month. Indeed, by now I had acquired quite a reasonable clientele, mainly through word-of-mouth recommendations. I had learned a great deal about sex, the male psyche, and the know-how of pleasing men—and women.

To show you how I looked after my people, my original client, Dirk, was still a good customer and had recommended me to some of his friends.

With me it wasn't the all-American wham-bam, thank you, ma'am. I really enjoyed my work, and I loved sex. I seldom faked my pleasure and never rushed my client.

Pearl could see everyone was pleased with me, and in time I insisted on having exclusively $50 dates, out of which I paid her $20. So my clientele became better quality, and instead of sales representatives, I started having company presidents, stockbrokers, lawyers, and real-estate men. But I was also outgrowing Pearl's nickel-and-dime downtown operation, and I knew I had to move up through the ranks to a better establishment.

Around November the change came through an introduction by one of my customers to two women who were to become very vital in my life for the next year. Their first names were Madeleine and Georgette, and they were two of the top madams in New York.

A horny guy named Jim Watney, who liked to sleep with ten girls at one time and once came with seven of them, phoned the madams and literally told them "Xaviera is a girl you can't do without."

Madeleine was, over the last few years, known to be the biggest madam in New York. She inherited the title from a lesbian lady called Daphne, whose brownstone on Lexington Avenue, complete with swimming pool and milk baths, was raided and closed down in June 1968. It made *Daily News* headlines, and that is the last thing a whorehouse needs. Councilman Carter Burden now occupies the premises for his political activities.

Madeleine's operation almost rivaled Daphne's for grandeur and size. Her five-bedroom house was a brownstone in the Murray Hill district and contained three floors of bedrooms, with another floor for bar, relaxation, and mingling.

It was a cold night in November when I was brought to her house to make up the number of girls required for a group of rich executives wanting to be entertained after a stag dinner at 21. Jim Watney and I rang the bell and waited several minutes before all the protection locks and devices were released to open the door. We were shown inside by a butler.

Wow, I never imagined Pearl's was a palace, but this place made her house look like an igloo.

The entrance was an elegant foyer with slate and marble tile floors and a magnificent chandelier. To the right was a living room lined with smoky mirrors. A rosewood dining table and a huge gourmet kitchen were visible in the background. Inside the room were nine or ten girls, all well dressed, and it looked more like a high-class model agency than a brothel.

Then I met Madeleine. She floated across the room in her Pucci gown, a woman in her late thirties, elegant, handsome, her makeup and hair immaculate.

"Welcome to my house, Xaviera," she said, and I was in for another surprise. That foreign accent! New York's reigning madam was from a country where I had lived, South Africa.

By way of introduction, Madeleine gave me a guided tour up the staircase from the entrance hall to the first floor, which had simply but tastefully furnished bedrooms to the left and right. The second floor was identical, differing only in colors.

The third floor was where the men would relax in between their activities. It was a big, beautiful, baronial room, very masculine, with beamed ceilings and heavy wooden benches. On one side there was a fully equipped bar, and on the other there was a cinema-size movie projector set up.

The butler, Felipe, saw to it that the men were helped in and out of their coats and shown to the bar or the other public rooms.

Overseeing the bedroom activity was Madeleine's red-haired young lesbian secretary, Cynthia, who wore a little black-and-white uniform and walked around keeping score of who went with whom and how many times. It is one of the hazards of this business that girls can claim they did more work than they did if there is not some kind of surveillance on them. On the other hand, a customer could claim he did less than he did. Either way, you would be cheated out of money. So Cynthia, who has since come to work for me as a call girl, kept score, and Madeleine arranged the pairings and acted charmingly to her clients.

This was my first contact with working girls as a group, and frankly I was apprehensive about mixing at first. I always imagined hookers as a breed were tough street types or brainless little runaway girls. Not so with Madeleine's girls. They were well groomed, attractive, and reasonably well educated.

As we waited for our customers, I wondered what does one sit around and talk about with a bunch of prostitutes. What kind of small talk can you make? Something like: What do you think of the Pentagon Papers? Or: Will the wage-and-price freeze affect prostitution? Or even: How's tricks? I didn't feel that it was in good taste to talk shop about money, johns, and so on, but being always curious about what makes people tick, I decided to conduct a little Harris Poll of my own. Where are you from, how long have you been doing this, do you enjoy sex in general, do you enjoy professional sex? In other words, I was asking them the eternal question: "What's a girl like you doing in a place like this?"

Carmen, the fiery Brazilian, said, "I hate this business, but my guy beats the hell out of me when I don't bring money home."

Crista, the German, cooed, "I am married, and my husband knows what I'm doing, and we like the extra income."

Sunny, the American, hissed, "I hate men. I am a lesbian; this is just a living to me."

There was one very pretty young girl who said that she did not mind her work; she merely used her earnings to pay her college tuition.

Nobody admitted liking what they were doing except me and one other girl, the Negro, Laura.

"Yes, I like sex, I like men. I like every bit of it as long as they don't give me a hard time." She laughed. Her voice was without the trace of hardness or bitterness in the other girls.

Laura and I immediately became friends. We both prospered

and later kept running into each other, either on jobs or on vacation. She became a high-class courtesan working on her own, and my own success you already know.

Finally the group of about ten or twelve slightly polluted young men, all dressed in black tie, showed up after their formal dinner, and were received by Felipe, the butler, who helped them out of their coats. Cynthia showed them to the bar, where they were given drinks and mingled with the girls until they made their choice or Madeleine made it for them.

Each man selected two girls, either separately or together, and everything went off smoothly. It was a night when business was an unmitigated pleasure.

They were all accommodated while Cynthia walked around the house dressed in her neat uniform, keeping score of who went in the green room, who went in the blue room, and who went in the red room, and with whom.

Around three in the morning, when everyone was content, dressed, and sitting around the downstairs dining room drinking coffee, Madeleine decided the evening had gone so well that she would put on a special late-late show as a bonus.

She had noticed that Laura and I hit it off very well together and were enthusiastic about our work, so she felt we should do a double striptease together on the big oak dining table.

I ought to have jumped at the chance to make it with Laura. However, there were reservations—I had never been with a Negro before, and my South African background made me slightly uptight.

Laura, however, had no such inhibitions, and when she peeled the clothes off that dynamite body with those big, brown breasts with nipples like ebony thimbles, I decided she would be my first black lover.

Madeleine put on some exciting music, and Laura and I commenced a sensual dance on top of the table. Laura was slowly undressing me, and as I watched her beautiful, black hips swaying before me, I got so hot that I started kissing her navel, and then I made my way down to her pussy. I caressed her buttocks, her legs, her hips, enjoying her velvet-soft skin. I brushed my lips against her pussy and then got back on my feet and moved behind her. I smoothed her hair away from her face and covered her neck and back with tiny bites. I could hear gasps from our overheated public, but I turned her to face me and sucked her nipples, which stood as inviting as cherries. I had pushed my leg between hers, and I could feel her juices flowing over me, so once more I went down and did not let up on her purple clitoris. The men and girls were gaping, as I spread wide her labia so that they all could see her great, wet, pink cunt, surrounded by black, springy hair.

The watching girls and guests came back to life, and pretty soon everyone was tearing off his clothes. Ties, pants, and shirts were flying around the room, and men were jerking off, and jumping on or under the table with girls. Even the madam herself became too excited to keep her clothes on and did a quick peel. I must say for almost forty she looked very attractive naked, with her big boobs sticking out like rocks because of a silicone job, as she climbed on the table and helped herself to a good-looking man.

One thing I learned about Madeleine was that if she wanted a particular man, which is the privilege of a madam, and he rejected her, she would become furious and take her anger out on everyone around her. But happily that night there was no such drama, and we all ended up in a big profitable gang bang, with a harried Cynthia running around trying to keep score of who came and who caused it.

That spontaneous swing made the house and the girls a lot of extra money, and Madeleine was justifiably happy with me the first night, because I started it all.

Before I went home, she invited me to be one of her regular girls. Around the same time I also met Georgette Harcourte, who had an establishment in a multistoried apartment building on York Avenue. Georgette was younger, very temperamental, and not quite so organized as Madeleine. But I learned early that you don't jump around from madam to madam. If you are getting good work with one, you had better stay with her.

I preferred Madeleine's because she had a more sophisticated, longer-established house with a better class of clients.

Both Georgette and her reasonably large operation were less reliable than Madeleine's. She was always moving from one place to another. Her living room was usually packed with cartons and looked a mess. And, what's more, she was not half the lady, nor did she have the savoir faire of Madeleine.

On being taken into Madeleine's stable, I severed all professional relationships with Pearl, although I kept in touch with her as a friend, because I liked the girl.

Also, at the time my professional life was accelerating, my straight life was falling apart at the seams. Things were getting hot at the office. My coworkers and employer were wondering why I was looking so tired, always getting masses of phone calls, and dressed generally far better than some little secretary on a lower-echelon income.

It was only a matter of time before the pennies dropped, and they got an open line on my activity. As would be appropriate at a consulate, my superior suggested diplomatically I would be better off working somewhere else. He even advised me of an available position at a United Nations mission, and gave me a good reference.

I took the suggestion, knowing that there was little alternative, and went through a series of multilingual typing and translating tests at the foreign mission. I was hired and started work
on November 1, 1969. The job was administrative, but almost as
dull as the one I had left, and it was just as well, because I wasn't
up to concentrating much effort or energy taking dictation from
my boss, the horny little ambassador, after a hard night's work.

I no longer wanted to stay in the apartment I had taken over
from Sonia; it was too far from my work. So around the time I
took the new job, I found a studio apartment near First Avenue
in the lower Fifties, five minutes' walk from the office.

Something happened during my move from one apartment
to the other that started reinforcing my feelings that in an illicit
profession like prostitution you are vulnerable to all kinds of
harassment. First the phony policeman, and now a nuisance
named Murray the Mover.

Murray the Mover was a big bear of a Turkish Jew who had
more in mind than moving my belongings, and persisted in a
conversation which I found irritating at the time, but in view of
subsequent events was somewhat significant.

"I bet you're a girl who likes fun and games, Miss Xaviera,"
Murray said with an ill-concealed smirk after the last piece of
furniture was out of the service elevator.

"Murray," I replied coldly, "what I like happens to be none of
your business."

"Don't be too upset, lady," he went on, "because I could help
a girl like you out in a lot of different ways."

"I don't see how I can use you except to get this furniture out
of the hallway. Otherwise I can pretty well help myself."

But Murray the Mover had more to say, and after his assistants were dismissed, he still hung around.

"This sure is a beautiful location for your line of work, miss," he said.

"Just what do you mean by that?"

"I happen to know this is a cool building, and you can work here as a hooker as long as you like. Just make sure you take care of the doormen."

"Okay, Murray, groovy." I didn't admit anything, and really wanted to get rid of him, but I was intrigued.

"You look like you're new in the business, fresh and natural. Stay that way. Be careful you don't get yourself into any trouble, because this can be a rough racket. But if you do, give me a call." He handed me a square of paper with his name and number scribbled on it.

"Fine, Murray. I hope I'll never need your help, but thanks anyway. Good-bye now, I've got work to do." Murray the Mover left, and I straightened up my studio for the coming night's business.

Life was well organized and ran smoothly for the next couple of months, although my job at the mission was even less agreeable than that at the consulate. I was made to feel like an "office foreigner," even though I could speak their language. And sometimes they would lapse into a national dialect to exclude me from conversations. Still, the atmosphere didn't bother me too much, as my professional night life was becoming more important, more active, and more profitable than the day job.

I could even manage to run home during lunch hours and turn a couple of tricks in my studio, or sometimes Madeleine or even Georgette would call up and ask me could I handle a midday quickie.

I had told Madeleine about the perverse, sexual fights I had had with my ex-fiancé and suggested that she might like me to take over the bondage and slave and master scenes. She agreed, and before long I had acquired an interesting collection of riding whips and paddles, which I used to good effect on my masochistic clients—who paid considerably more than the straight guys for the privilege. I would ask Madeleine to try to give me advance notice so I could at least wear the appropriate clothing, such as a leather jacket or skirt, black turtleneck sweater, or something else tough- or vicious-looking, and save the time of changing during the lunch hour.

One thing I liked about doing jobs for Madeleine was the discreet way she asked me on the office phones. "Xaviera, I've got a Scotch [meaning $50 customer] or a champagne [meaning $100]; will you be available for a drink around noon or one P.M.?"

She would often crack up because she had never known a little secretary who made a few hundred extra dollars a week during her lunch hours. The idea of my running down and performing a complex slave scene amused her even more.

However, some of my customers were not so diplomatic when they called up, which is what led to the beginning of the end of my new job. My biggest problem at the mission turned out to be the aging spinster switchboard operator, who, I later learned, listened in on all my calls. And some of them weren't what one would call very subtle. "Xaviera," they would say, "I want to get laid at one P.M. Meet you at your house. Okay?"

The fifty-year-old spinster didn't suspect it was for money, and started spreading the talk that Mademoiselle Xaviera was "the greatest *courtisane* of the *mission permanente de Nations Unies. Scandale! Horrible!*"

I sensed imminent disaster in the air and figured the only way to save my head was to seduce the horny little ambassador. If the heat really was on, it would help to have him on my side.

On a Friday afternoon, the bespectacled ambassador came to my place for drinks and, in his mind, a slow continental-type love scene. But I couldn't spare the time for romance that day because a couple of stockbrokers were expected around 7:00 P.M.

I poured the ambassador a cognac and sat him on the sofa. "Xaviera," he began, "how long I have dreamed of this moment." As he launched on a tale of romance, and desire, I removed his coat, tie, shirt, and shoes, and by the time he got around to how he was going to gently kiss my hair, my eyes, my throat—ad nauseam—he was clad only in his birthday suit.

I quickly made love to him, giving him my best efforts, considering the time available. He must have enjoyed it, because for the next couple of weeks, as I sat on his knee taking dictation, he would ask me, "Xaviera, are you free for an hour after work?" He would have had cardiac arrest if I told him I was rarely free these days, but I didn't charge him, so he didn't know the truth. "Oh, Mr. Ambassador," I would answer, "you're invited to my place this evening at six."

Things, however, were getting so unfriendly at the office that soon not even his intervention could help me. Certain staff members, whipped along by the narrow-minded spinster—who was by now getting wise—demanded an investigation into my ability to dress so well on a secretary's salary, and the meaning of all the "obscene" phone calls.

One morning when I breezed into work, my desk had been opened, and my little address book, which I stupidly kept in the office, had been commandeered. So, within three months of starting at the mission, my legitimate life as a secretary was over forever.

Six

Shakedown

9 was still working at the United Nations mission when I discovered what a vicious racket there is in New York in blackmailing vulnerable girls and married women who might try to make some extra money in prostitution. These blackmailers are even more dangerous to part-time hookers than the police.

I was living in my new studio apartment in the low East Fifties when the blackmailers, who had obviously been watching me for some time, paid me a call.

It was a raw, cold evening toward the end of November when I came home from the office and found an envelope stuck under my door. My first thought, when I opened the door and stooped down to pick up the envelope, was that it was a rent notice from the landlord. It was only three weeks since that hood moving man, Murray, had put my furniture in the apartment, and as yet I had not paid my rent besides the deposit.

My name was written on the envelope in very scribbly, more or less childish, uncontrolled handwriting, with a pencil, not a pen. I opened the envelope as I walked in and took my coat off. And all of a sudden an intuitive feeling told me that this envelope contained dangerous news for me.

Only one thing came out of the envelope: a Polaroid picture, which shocked me tremendously. Someone had put the pictures, which Mac the so-called cop (who I later learned was a phony) stole from my old apartment, into a group and took this Polaroid shot of them. There I was in one photo sucking a huge cock, and in the others, playing with myself. There was no letter with the pictures.

I was badly scared and immediately ran out of the apartment and took the elevator down to the lobby. I went up to the doorman on duty and said to him, "Listen, I'm in trouble." I trusted this doorman. He was a kind of fatherly type.

He knew I was hooking, of course, but I was paying him off. I didn't show him the picture or tell him exactly what had happened. I just said that some person came up to my apartment and put an envelope under the door which shouldn't have been put there.

"Did you see anyone going up unannounced?" I asked.

The doorman scratched his head and finally said, "Let me think. Yes, now that you ask me, I remember seeing a young guy this afternoon. I thought he must be drunk or doped up. I don't know what those kids take nowadays, but he couldn't walk straight. He needed a shave, his clothes were dirty and ragged." The doorman frowned to himself. "He was a young punk with long, stringy blond hair hanging in his face, and he said he had something to deliver to you."

The doorman grinned now. "He mispronounced your name

something awful, so I told him I'd take the message to you. But he said he wanted to deliver it himself, and he would just push it under your door. So finally I let him go up."

I couldn't think of anyone who answered the description, but I thanked the doorman, gave him five dollars, and went back to my apartment. I knew this was no joke, and as though to confirm this thought, the telephone rang. The voice on the other end was heavy with that low-class New York accent. It said, "Miss Xaviera?"

I knew the call had to do with the pictures. "Yes," I whispered.

"So, Miss Xaviera, I hope you found your letter."

"Yes," I said, trying to stop my voice from quivering.

"Honey, you'd better think our proposition over very seriously, and we want an answer by Wednesday. In fact, we are going to call you tomorrow night at seven." This was already Monday. "We expect you to have five thousand dollars ready for us, or else . . ."

Upon which I said, "What do you mean? Five thousand dollars for those pictures?"

In a sneering voice the man said, "Yeah. We know you don't have your immigration papers. We can get your sexy little ass kicked out of the country in forty-eight hours by proving to the immigration department that you are posing for pornographic pictures." He had a mean laugh.

"We can give the pictures to the people where you work, and you'll be fired and be in big trouble with immigration. Think about it. We'll be back in touch tomorrow at seven."

The man hung up, and in my life I never remember being so upset. I had been on my own for less than a year since Carl left. Apart from Sonia, I didn't have any real friends because of the wild life I had been leading. I knew some lawyers and influential men who were customers, but all of a sudden I was faced with the problem of raising $5,000. I looked through my address book wondering whom I could call.

For about four months I had been dating a sweet, conservative young lawyer named Martin Joffe. He had seen my suffering after my break with Carl, and was very upset after I met Pearl by what he regarded as the downfall of a nice Dutch girl. He was a tender, loving friend on whom I could always rely, and I was very fond of him. So he was the first person I called, but he had no solution. He warned me against paying anything to a blackmailer.

"Once you start," he warned, "you can never get him off your back."

I tried to borrow $5,000 from my rich clients, assuring them that if necessary I would give up my job and screw my way out of debt, but it was brought home to me that the last thing that they wanted was to become involved in a prostitute's private problems.

So I was on the phone all night, and nobody helped me out.

The next morning I was on the verge of a nervous breakdown, when I found in my pocketbook, just before leaving for the office, the piece of paper on which Murray the Mover had written his name and phone number.

I remembered how he had known instinctively that I was working as a prostitute even though I had a daytime job. Murray, being a mover, wasn't exactly a sweet pussycat, and I thought this was precisely the time to call a rough boy instead of all those nice, sophisticated jet-set people who are full of promises they do not live up to. I called Murray just before leaving for work and explained what had happened. He said if this blackmailer was going to call me tonight at seven, he would be at my apartment at six-thirty. Murray told me not to have any dates and not to plan on going anywhere until this thing was settled. "I just want you to be with me, and that you will do what I tell you—that's all."

This was an order, and right after five o'clock I went home. I had made a date at nine-thirty that night with a lawyer from Canada to go to dinner, and I had no way to reach him. He was recommended to me by my stockbroker, and when I called Wall Street, my broker didn't know how to find the lawyer. I just had no way to cancel this date.

I was home before six and canceled every person I was supposed to see that night, and I was so nervous I barked at the men who called me on the phone. "Leave me alone; don't bother me for the rest of the night."

At six-thirty sharp, Murray rang the doorbell. I had not seen him since he moved me in three weeks before. He is a very tough-looking man and has a dark, pockmarked face and bushy black hair.

Murray seemed nervous himself when he came in. He looked around my studio apartment, first into the bathroom, where I had a phone so I could call people while I was in the tub. He said this was good, and as he looked around, he was talking.

"Xaviera, I want you to do exactly what I tell you. If anything happens tonight, we will be together. Just don't be afraid. I know what I'm doing."

Murray told me not to be frightened, but I *was* frightened and trying to keep from shaking. I was not really intending to do anyone—even Mac, who stole the pictures—any harm. All I wanted was to have a man with me when I met the people who were blackmailing me; somebody powerful who would maybe smack them on the nose a little and say, "Listen, give the pictures back to the girl and stop the bullshit!"

"Okay," Murray said, "now remember, usually blackmailers are not there to hurt you, they just want money, that's all. When they call at seven, you answer in the bathroom, and I'll pick up in the living room. We'll pretend that I'm your uncle. The only living relative you have in this country. I'm representing you, see? I have a car, and if they want to meet us we'll meet them."

Exactly at seven o'clock the telephone rang. I answered, and it was the guy who asked me for the money the night before. Murray picked up in the living room, and with the door open I could see him from the bathroom. He was nervous, too. I told the man that my uncle was with me and would handle the matter.

Then Murray started talking. "Hello, this is Mr. Arkstein. I'm Miss Xaviera's uncle and only living relative she's got here. I'm representing the girl. I know it is a very bad thing you found those pictures of her. I don't want my niece to be deported."

Murray really sounded like a meek, worried uncle. "Tell me how much you want, and we'll meet you," he went on. "I want to meet you tonight and get this thing over with, because the girl didn't sleep last night, and I don't want her to go through any more of this aggravation."

Finally the man said, "Okay. We want five thousand dollars. We will meet you in front of the monument entrance to the Queens Cemetery at eight o'clock tonight." It was past seven already.

Murray agreed, and after we hung up he said to me, "Xaviera, why don't you get me a beer? I've got to make a phone call."

I went into the kitchen and poured Murray's beer, and came back just in time to hear the last part of the conversation, which sounded more or less in code. I heard him say, "Be ready to pick up the bag of potatoes at the monument in the cemetery in Queens at eight-fifteen."

I didn't know what he meant, but I was petrified with fright, because it sounded like gangster talk. Murray drank his beer, and at ten minutes after seven he said, "Okay, let's get moving. The car's outside."

"What's going to happen, Murray?" I asked. It was a horrible, cold, sleeting, and raining night. No way did I want to go out.

Murray said, "Xaviera, do what I tell you and don't ask questions. We'll drive out to Queens, and I'll tell you about myself on the way. Bring your umbrella."

I took my umbrella along; it had a long spike at the end. We left the apartment. My hands were perspiring, something that never happened to me before. I was perspiring all over, and I never in my whole life have experienced so much nervous tension as that night. Out on the street we got into this old, smashed-up car.

"Couldn't we go in a better car, Murray?" I asked.

He told me not to worry, and we started out for Queens. It was pouring rain, and we could hardly see through the windshield. I don't know how Murray found the way. And as we drove, Murray told me some things about himself.

"Xaviera, you should know that I'm not only a mover. I'm involved in many other things. I'm sure you've heard about the Mafia. I work with them."

I started to tremble when he said the word.

"What do you mean, the Mafia?" I practically shouted. "I don't want to get involved with the Mafia!"

I had seen movies and read about the Mafia, how people get killed and disappear from the face of the earth. And up till then I had been so careful not to get involved with the Mafia.

"I've done ten years in jail," Murray went on. "I'm thirty-seven years old now. I have survived so far, and now I'm sticking my neck way out, taking a lot of risks, but I hate to see a nice little girl like you getting pushed around and in trouble."

He turned from the windshield and looked straight at me. "I'm doing this for you, but you've got to do one thing for me. This is no kid's game we're in. This is dangerous, serious work tonight. You've got to do just what I say every minute, and you'll be all right. Don't be afraid, and do exactly as I tell you."

I think my eyes were as wide as the ocean. "What do you mean, Murray?" I asked.

"I'll tell you, Xaviera. Whatever you see tonight, you'll forget. And don't ever mention my name or tell anybody what happened."

I looked out the car window at the wet streets and the rain, and I was cold, yet perspiring at the same time.

"Murray," I asked after a while, "why do we have to meet in front of a cemetery in Queens, of all places, which is a very scary place, especially on a gloomy night like this?"

Murray answered me as though I was a dumb child. "Xaviera," he said, "that's the idea! What do you think? They're going to meet you in front of Saks Fifth Avenue? Or in front of Maxwell's Plum? They've got to meet us where there will be no witnesses."

At fifteen after eight Murray stopped in front of the cemetery. There was a highway right next to us with traffic buzzing by. To our right was the monument, and beside it, with an arched roof, a little dead-end alley maybe fifteen feet long.

There was no other car to be seen when we parked. "Murray," I said, "this can't be right. It's a quarter after eight, and why aren't they here?" I wanted to go home in the worst way before something terrible happened.

Murray looked at me fiercely. "Do as I tell you. Get in the back of the car and shut up. And for Christ's sake, don't shake like that, like some little bird freezing to death."

So I took my umbrella, my weapon for the evening, and climbed over the front seat and sat in the back of the car. But nothing happened. We saw cars drive by, and nobody stopped. The rain kept pouring down, and I was freezing. Murray smoked one cigarette after another, and I saw he was getting more and more nervous. He opened the window.

Then slowly, from nowhere, a car pulled up behind us with its lights on. "Murray, they're here," I said. Looking out the back window, I could see that there were *two* men in the front seat of the car. "Murray, that's unfair," I said. "We talked to only one man."

Murray kept saying, "Don't worry, don't worry." The car pulled up and passed us, and we could see the men looking into our car to see how many of us there were. Then the car kept going and stopped about four car lengths in front of us. The two men lit cigarettes and smoked them. Then a fellow stepped out of the car and came close to us. Under the streetlight, I could see he was dressed in a white rain jacket and blue jeans. He had long, stringy blond hair and a three- or four-day-old beard. He was definitely a punky guy and looked exactly like the description of the person who put the note under my door. He knocked on the window next to Murray, who cranked it down and said, "Hiya. I'm her uncle."

The guy said, "Can I talk to you, buddy?"

Murray opened the door on the passenger side, and the untidy-looking guy walked around the car. He was talking and babbling to himself, and he finally got in. Obviously he was high on acid.

His eyes were sort of rolling around in his head, and he started saying things like, "We don't mean so badly, but girls like this shouldn't be around, dragging dirty pictures around to show everybody."

I got aggravated and shouted, "What do you mean, show them to everybody? Those pictures were stolen out of my apartment!"

"Shut up!" Murray said to me, and I shut my mouth. Then he turned to this junkie beside him. "Let's go outside and talk. Who is the guy up front in the car?"

The doped-up hippie type said, "None of your business, man. I'm going to go away. We're ready to take four thousand. Let's settle right now."

Murray shook his head. "No. I don't think we should settle it right now. Let's go outside and not discuss it in front of this lady."

He gestured to me to open the window just a little so that I could hear what was happening, and in the pouring rain Murray stepped out on his side of the car, and the other guy got out as well. I don't think he knew if it was raining or the sun was shining, the way he was babbling.

The minute Murray left the car, the man in the car up front got out, too. He opened an umbrella and walked up to Murray and the doped-up kid. He acted like the leader, and although the light was bad, especially with the umbrella over his head, I could almost swear it was Mac. The same big, fat-looking type. The three of them talked for about ten minutes, when all of a sudden two big, strong headlights illuminated the scene. A truck stopped behind us.

When the lights hit us, I was more scared than ever, if that is possible. What the hell was happening? Were people trying to kill us, or what? But the truck driver just stepped out of the cab, and for the first time I saw there was a telephone booth there. The driver went to the booth and made a call. It seemed like he was in there for an hour, but in reality it was maybe two minutes.

All the time I wondered what Murray and Mac and the junkie were talking about and what Murray was going to do. Finally the truck driver left the phone booth, and the truck pulled away.

Mac, holding the umbrella down over his head, went back to his car, got in, and closed the door after him. Then I saw Murray gesturing to the blond guy, and I could hear a few words he was saying. "Wait a minute. I'll get it for you."

Murray came back to the car and said in a loud voice, "I'm going to give him his goddamned four thousand and get your pictures back."

Like a little idiot I said, "But, Murray, I don't have four thousand dollars."

In a rasping whisper he said, "Shut up." And he reached in and took out a brown bag that looked like it was stuffed with something. He straightened up and gestured to the blond guy to go stand inside the covered-over dead-end alley, where he could count the money out of the rain and see that it was right.

I watched as Murray walked toward the alley, his back to me. The other guy stood with his face turned toward me, and I could see him through the rain, somewhat blurred. Then I saw Murray reaching into the bag as though to start giving the money to the kid. Next thing I knew there were three very soft pops, and the young boy collapsed on the ground. Nobody but me could see into the alley, and then Murray walked back to the car at normal speed and shoved something into his pocket. He got into the car, and we drove away. I was still sitting in the back seat.

"My God, Murray, what did you do?" I asked.

As usual, he just said, "Don't worry."

"But how can I help worrying?" I said. "Murray, you just shot a man three times. I heard you shoot him with a silencer on your gun. Was that what you had in the bag?" I kept asking questions as we drove back toward New York.

Finally Murray said, "We don't take halfway measures with bastards like these. What right do they have to blackmail a hard-working girl like you?"

"But Murray, you still don't have the pictures," I pointed out.

All the way back to New York, Murray didn't say anything except, "Don't worry, I'll deliver the pictures tomorrow." But in my mind I kept seeing this young boy slowly collapse and fall in the alley.

Okay, he was a head, a useless junkie. But I saw him lying there. He was still a human being, although used in a dirty business by his boss, who got away scot-free. So I kept insisting, "Murray, please tell me what happened so far."

Finally he said, "That jerk in the front seat didn't see or hear me shoot the kid because I had a silencer on my gun. There's a lot of work to do tonight. I've got to get rid of the gun."

"But what about the big shot in the front seat?" I asked. I was still worrying about getting my pictures back.

"He'll be taken care of, too," Murray said, staring out the windshield at the wet street.

"He's going to be killed, too?" I tried to keep my voice low.

"That's about it," Murray said. "Two of my boys were hiding behind the cemetery walls."

He laughed harshly. "Those finks couldn't pick a sweeter place—for me. In about ten or fifteen minutes that slughead in the front seat will wonder where his hopped-up friend is, and when he goes to look for him . . ." Murray laughed again.

"When he sees his buddy lying in the alley, my two guys will grab him. And what happens after that, I'll tell you tomorrow."

At nine-twenty Murray left me off in front of my apartment and said he would see me tomorrow. I went up to my apartment just in time to answer the bell, when this straight lawyer I had a date with came around. Here I had been going through the most scary hours of my life, and this lawyer comes in fresh and peppy and says, "Hi, how are you? Nice to meet you!"

I could hardly talk. We went down to Chinatown to a restaurant. I dropped my plate on the floor before I got down half a spoon of wonton soup.

Finally I told the guy, "Listen, I'm so shook up about something, I can't tell you. Take me to a hotel. Fuck me. Do whatever you want, but don't take me home. I don't want to go home. I'm not even going to work tomorrow."

I told him part of the terrifying story, but naturally suppressed the murder. He was very understanding and took me to his room, where he did not even try to fuck me but tucked a hundred-dollar bill into my purse.

The next morning at eleven o'clock, the lawyer dropped me off in front of my house. I was just about to walk up to my apartment building when I saw Murray in his moving van. There was a big smile on his face, and an envelope in his hands. I went over to him, and he took the pictures out. There were all the pictures Mac had stolen that night.

"Murray," I said, "come up and tell me what happened." So Murray came up, we had some coffee, and he told me everything.

Right after he left me off, he had to dispose of the gun. Meanwhile, the two Mafia guys at the cemetery grabbed Mac as he was leaning over his dead partner.

"Listen, buddy," they said, "if you don't show us the place where the pictures of the girl are, then you'll end up like your pal here, dead. Right?"

Mac got in their car and took them to some shabby apartment in Queens. Murray's guys found thousands of pictures of different girls they had been blackmailing for the last year or two.

Mac was so scared that he gave them my pictures immediately.

But Murray and his Mafia guys weren't content just to get my pictures back. These blackmailers were working without what you might call a franchise from the Mafia godfather in Queens.

They made Mac tell them who was behind this whole blackmail syndicate, and he was so scared he said, "Okay, it's a lawyer."

Mac took them to this lawyer, and then Murray's hoods grabbed him, too, and three people were taken care of in total.

The two Mafia guys and Murray had to dispose of three bodies that same night.

This is what Murray told me, and obviously I realized that I had to compensate these guys for their services. At least it wouldn't be $5,000.

But in the meantime, I was being so stupid and such an idiot that after Murray told me all this and showed me he had my pictures back, I said, "Murray, I don't want those pictures in the house anymore. I don't want them. You get rid of them for me." So far he hadn't asked for any money. But eventually Murray charged me $2,000 for services rendered.

And, of course, this morning was not the last time I was to see Murray. Just a few weeks later he came back to see me and suggested I ought to "invest" my money with him. By lending it, I would get back more in a couple of months.

I could see he wasn't *asking* me if I wanted to make an investment, he was telling me I had to. I was making money by then, having left the U.N. job to go full-time into the business, so I gave Murray $2,000. He said he would put it in the street for me—shylock it. He explained it would mean making 5 to 10 percent interest on the money each week and, of course, getting the original sum back in a short time. Naturally I let myself forget I was dealing with somebody who was involved with many very bad people and who was, even though he helped me, a pretty shady character himself.

After I gave the money to Murray, I waited each week for some payment on interest, but nothing happened except that Murray kept coming around for freebies and gave me excuses why he didn't have my money. Finally, when I started to be insistent with Murray, he said, "Look, Xaviera, don't worry. You'll get your money. Just don't bug me. Remember what happened to those jerks that bugged you?"

The message was very clear. Now the problem was to stop Murray from coming around. I would gladly have given him another thousand if I never had to see him again. I was almost as worried about getting involved with Murray and his people as I was about the pictures. He even was sending friends to me and telling me to be nice to them. They were creeps, and I almost got sick every time he called.

And then the F.B.I. approached me.

I was still in the same Fifty-first Street studio when the doorbell rang. The doorman called up and said the F.B.I. wanted to see me. I was terrified, even though the murder—or maybe fake murder—had happened three months before.

So into my apartment came this nice-looking F.B.I. agent, Bill Tillman. He seemed to be a pleasant-type Irishman, but remembering Mac, the fake cop, I asked him if he could please identify himself. He was indeed F.B.I., very nice, and then he showed me a picture of Murray and asked me if I knew the person whose picture he was holding up.

I almost fainted. I really thought, Xaviera, this is it. You're going to hang, you're going to get the electric chair, they've found out you got that kid killed and are involved in a triple murder. But somehow I kept my composure.

You don't fool around with F.B.I. people, so I said, "Yes, I know him. He is Murray the moving man." Then I asked this F.B.I. man, "Why are you looking for Murray?"

Bill said they had followed his steps and found out that a couple of months ago he was at my place quite often in the afternoons.

"We're looking for this man because he's killed about eight people so far that we know about," Bill told me. "He's involved with fraud, hijacking, bootlegging, white slavery, and any other illegal thing you can imagine. What is your connection with him?"

Of course I wasn't going to tell him exactly what had happened and that I was a prostitute, but I was stupid enough not to take the phone off the hook, and it kept ringing. I had to answer it, so he quickly got the idea.

"Have you had any bad experiences with this man?" Bill asked.

I told him that I shylocked $2,000 with Murray and hadn't even been paid back any interest. Bill said I could whistle for my money, and I'd better not ever see Murray again.

Just as he was leaving, the F.B.I. man said, "We are not after prostitutes, but just don't let us catch you fooling around with girls underage or violating the Mann Act." At that time I had been in the business only about five months, so I didn't know about those things. But I asked some friends, and now I'm very careful not to have a girl under eighteen working for me.

Once I took a girlfriend down to Miami for convention work, but I made her buy her own ticket, and we left on separate planes. That way nobody can say *I'm* transporting girls over state lines for immoral purposes, which is the Mann Act.

Murray called me only one more time to tell me the F.B.I. was putting big heat on him, investigating every bar where he hung out, and he couldn't get my money loose. I was so thankful he was going away that I didn't care about losing the money. Then he told me something which relieved me more than anything else.

"Look, kid"—his voice was harsh in my ear—"there wasn't any killing out there at the cemetery. I scared those bums into putting on that show for you. I figured since you ain't gonna see me no more, you ought to know. When they found how well I was connected, they just melted away and gave me your pictures."

I wanted to believe him, I still want to believe him, and I think I do. But I remember the F.B.I. man telling me Murray had killed eight people, and I can still see the way the young blond guy sort of slid to the ground.

But from this experience I learned to be very careful about letting anybody get anything from me, and especially I have never let any pictures be taken any more of me sucking a cock or anything like that.

Seven

Arrests

9n my opinion, no brothel can operate more than a year in New York without being raided at least once by police.

I have been busted three times in my own house and once in the establishment of another madam, Georgette Harcourte. Each arrest is a serious nuisance, because all we want to do is get on with our work and not bother, or be bothered by, anybody else.

You can try protecting yourself by carefully screening your phone callers, making sure there is no money exchanged until the customer has participated, or by using police locks to keep out police. I have special code words with my customers.

But no matter how careful you are or how many precautions you take, if they want to penetrate you, so to speak, they can always find a way. The new no-knock laws make it easier for them to push their way in legally, and they don't need search warrants to seize your books and telephones.

The methods, reasons, and penalties for arrest are as different as they are sometimes ridiculous.

A neighbor can report you for disturbance, a rival madam can report you to cripple the competition, or an irrational customer with some imagined grievance can yell police, which is, I believe, what happened to me the second time I got busted.

A little lunatic called Nicky, whom I threw out for bugging my girls and upsetting my clients, ran down to the local police precinct and filed a complaint.

"They're running a whorehouse up there, and they don't want to service me," he told them.

But the police busted me and dug into all my financial business, came up with a Dun and Bradstreet triple-A rating, and told the judge I was the biggest madam operating in New York City today. It looked bad for a while, but my lawyer got the charge reduced to a misdemeanor, and in the end I got off with a $100 fine. Plus a staggering legal fee, naturally.

The arrest before that happened in my house, too, and I admit it was partly through my own carelessness, because I was too busy that night to check out a client's credentials. Normally I would ask a caller to prove he is a customer by identifying something in my house or describing to me the girl he saw last time. Or, if he is new, to give me another client's name as a reference. But this night a guy named Artie called, said he was from Brooklyn and that he was a friend of "Mr. Roberts."

Well, that usually would not be a sufficient recommendation, because I know about six Mr. Robertses. But he sounded very charming, and also you can say I might have been a little greedy, because he wanted to bring along another three customers.

They arrived about an hour later, and the bedrooms were

full, and a couple of guys were ahead of them, but they didn't mind waiting.

They were a happy bunch of guys—one Jewish, one Irish, and two Italians—they had a drink and sat around and talked and joked.

Meantime, they asked me to send out for three other girls for them, which I was happy to do. The girls arrived, then one of the men flashed a badge and identified himself, after pushing me his fee in advance.

"Hey, pussycat," he said, "we're not exactly what you think we are; we're not johns." Which amazed me, because they had pretty authentic hard-ons in their pants, each with a girl on his lap. "We're police officers, and you're under arrest."

This time my lawyer got me off with another hundred-dollar fine on reduced charges by proving this was entrapment.

Entrapment means that a police officer deliberately causes you to commit a crime, and he cannot then legally arrest you for it, which is fair.

Another method the police use to bust you is to wait downstairs and grab a client as he leaves and intimidate him into fingering you, so to speak.

They ask him if he has paid to get laid, and if he says, "No, I was just visiting my mother," they say, "Okay, we'll take your name and address and just let your wife know what a dutiful son you are." The guy gets frightened and tells all. Then they either bring him straight back and confront you, with your accuser, or they wait until more customers come in so they can catch you all together in the act.

This is the way I was busted, for the first time, in the house of Georgette Harcourte, and I still remember it as a very ugly and degrading experience.

At this time I was working mostly for Georgette, because Madeleine caught me passing my visiting cards around among her clients and she got furious. I felt bad about it, because Madeleine's was definitely the best house in town and had the most sophisticated clientele. Georgette's clients were mostly drunk stockbrokers and weirdos, and most of her girls were not very attractive. Also, I must point out that Georgette's 50–50 split was less fair than Madeleine's 60–40. Financially, Georgette was so tough that if you had to take a taxi from here to Timbuktu, she wouldn't give you a break. In her house the girls were never allowed to fix themselves a cold drink, much less have something to eat, even if they were there over four hours. In my house the girls can eat and drink what they want.

Still, Georgette's was where I was working, and she loved to have me because I was so hardworking, reliable, and resourceful. I was also the only girl who could get into the Plaza or Waldorf after midnight without difficulty. I would put on a conservative sweater and skirt, white socks and shoes, and fix my hair into pigtails. I hardly ever wear makeup, even to this day, now that I am a big madam, so I already had a fresh, natural look. I'd put a pair of glasses on my nose, and then I would hold a book under my arm and breeze in past the security men like a college girl. Before I knocked on the client's door I would undo my hair, remove my socks, take off my glasses, and throw the book in the trash can.

Another thing Georgette liked about me was that I could take care of the big cocks, any length, any width, because I love it.

So I was an asset for her house, and she knew she could call me any time of the day or night, and I'd run over for her.

This night in February 1970, Georgette called me to come over and help her with a stag party for a group of five investment bankers. I recall there was a blizzard going outside, and I was nearly frozen when I arrived at the Pavilion, where she had her penthouse. I was busy thawing my hands as I stepped from the elevator, but I noticed a little Chinese guy wearing dark glasses, who must have been her previous customer, leaving.

I went inside and was assigned to Carter Miles, a banker who is famous for his big penis that none of the other girls could take. They call him the Long Mile, for obvious reasons.

I remember Carter pounding away at me. He took forever to climax, as he was very drunk. His friends were all finished and getting dressed.

Meantime, I heard Georgette accept a phone booking for another two guys who were coming by, and she asked me to stay on for them. So everybody was dressed now except me.

I was just sitting, relaxing, one customer's head in my lap, when the doorbell buzzed. "Let me greet them in the nude," I jokingly said to Georgette. "What a wonderful reception that will be," one of the bankers mumbled.

I stood beside her as she undid half a dozen locks. She opened the door, and the two guys were there. Both very large men, one was bald and kind of vicious-looking, but I suppose they can't help being born ugly, and their money is as good as everybody else's. So I jumped forward and greeted them. "Hello, darling," I said to the big, bald one. "Come on in, let me take your jacket; make yourself at home." But whom did I notice behind them but the little Asian-looking guy in the dark glasses, whom they'd obviously grabbed on the way out, and the weasel was wetting his pants, he was so frightened.

The men flashed their badges and said, "Vice squad, you're all under arrest." Then everything happened at once, as eight uniformed cops burst through the door, and chaos broke loose.

The girls were screaming, the customers were having a fit, and only Marianna, Georgette's maid, kept her cool and hid the books. Even Georgette, the madam herself, was yelling stupid threats at the cops. This for me was a very scary moment, and I didn't know what was going to happen next.

Meanwhile, my own little black book with my clients all listed was in the next room with my clothes, and I was standing there naked. The first thing I instinctively did was run into the bedroom, rip out the pages with the addresses on them, and hide them underneath Georgette's laundry while the uniformed cops were turning the place over for drugs.

One came to the bathroom just as I finished hiding the pages and ordered me to get dressed to go with everyone to the station. But in all the disturbance, I couldn't find my bikini underpants, my panty hose, or my bra (which people were wearing in those days), so I had to go out into the freezing night with nothing under my coat but a light minidress.

The neighbors were lined up in the hall watching as they herded us out like geese into the squad cars and off to the precinct.

It seemed we were bumping and circling around the city for hours, and meanwhile the Irish cop beside me grabbed my hand and put it on his huge hard-on. The wagon was dark, my laugh was cynical.

"What *is* this nonsense?" I said at the top of my voice. "You arrest us for selling it, and now you want a freebie in the car!" This seemed such an inappropriate thing to do that I cracked up. "What the hell, we're going to prison, we might as well give it away," I said nervously.

The other girls were mortified. "Take it easy, Xaviera," they said; "this is a serious matter."

But to me this was the breaking point. We were being pushed around like common whores, we were upset, my ass was literally freezing off without my underpants, and this cop wanted to get his rocks off. Embarrassed, he shifted uneasily away from me, his ardor considerably cooled.

It was around 1:00 A.M. when we arrived at the precinct house, and we were again herded up a flight of filthy stairs and into a dirty office, where Lieutenant Greenleaf, the big, bald ape who arrested me, took off his coat and sat down at his desk.

We could make a couple of phone calls if we were quick about it, they told us, but the trouble was that I didn't have anyone to call except Paul Lindfeld, a jewelery designer I met in Miami whom I'd been going out with steadily since Christmas.

Even though it was late, I hoped he wouldn't mind helping me out, because he was my lover, after all.

"Paul," I said, "I'm awfully sorry to disturb you at this hour, but I am in some serious trouble. I've been arrested, I'm worried, I don't know what to do."

The last thing in the world I expected was his answer. "I don't want to know about it," he said. "Don't tell them you are calling me, don't mention my name, and scratch it out of your book in case they confiscate it."

It shows you how much you can sometimes depend on a man even when he claims to love you—when you need a helping hand, and there's nothing in it for him, he lets you down. What a do-gooder.

Time passed by very slowly at the police station, and nothing was happening for ages except that we were hungry and cold. Finally they decided to interrogate us one by one.

Georgette whispered in my ear "Deny you were paid," which turned out to be true, because we lost our pay for that night.

"And don't tell them who you are or where you live." When my turn came, a young Irish cop sat me down and asked my name. Despite Georgette's advice, I gave it to him. There was no alternative. "Address, age, and occupation?" he pursued. Occupation? This struck me as a redundant kind of question, so I answered, "Nymphomaniac." This big idiot asked, "How do you spell that?" "N-y-m-p-h—" I began, and the girls cracked up, and even two detectives dozing in chairs started laughing.

Despite the humor, I was depressed about this whole thing, and it was cold in there. I was very tired, so I climbed on a desk and tried to get some sleep. Behind me as I lay down I heard the cop interrogating Georgette, and they didn't have to ask her name, because she was already one of the most notorious madams in New York at that time.

"Hey, you're typing all kinds of errors on that sheet," I heard her say to him. So the cop replied, "Yeah, how can I concentrate?" He pointed at me. "Look at that broad there with her bare ass sticking out in my face."

Around 5:00 A.M. we were once again pushed into the squad cars, and this time we went downtown to the Tombs—my first visit—where we went through the whole rigamarole, filling in forms and making statements all over again. Only this was an even more horrible place than the station house—full of robbers, hoodlums, drunks, addicts, street fighters, and streetwalkers.

We had to get mug shots taken and submit to the most humiliating kind of physical examination by a big dyke-ish matron.

We had to bend backward, forward, and spread our legs so that if we carried anything in our vaginas it would most probably fall out. We were ordered to the bathroom whether we wanted to go or not, and then we were shoved into separate cells. People were talking, coughing, and vomiting, and there was a very grim atmosphere.

In the cell next to me, a black girl fifteen years old kept telling me in a whiny southern accent that she had been pushing drugs since she was twelve. She was dying for a cigarette, and she wouldn't leave me alone. One of our girls had some, so we passed them from hand to hand to shut up her dragging voice.

It was terribly cold on the benches, and that night passed slowly, fitfully, without any possibility of sleep. Around 8:00 A.M. we were taken to an even worse cell, full of vicious-looking black street hookers with long boots, colored wigs, and leather miniskirts. The horrible odor in there made me gasp; I tried not to breathe.

They started asking us all kinds of questions, as though we made a habit of spending our nights in these stinking jails. One black girl with bruises all over her face took an interest in me and wouldn't stop demanding information. She was one of those people who thump your arm when they want to know something.

"Hey," she said, "you with the blond hair!" *Thump*. "You must be high-priced jet-set call girls, the twenty-five-dollar-an-hour kind."

"No, I beg your pardon," I said, "we're *one hundred* dollars an hour." I was bragging, of course, but we felt like society ladies against those human dregs.

She didn't want to appear jealous, so she said, "Hey, sweetie"—nudge again—"hope you got your old man waiting outside to get you out." "What's an old man?" I asked, because I wasn't familiar with street-hooker terminology in those days. "A pimp, don't you have a pimp?" *Shove, push*.

She was really knocked out when I didn't know what a pimp

was, much less have one waiting outside. I wished she would shut up, because this talk was bugging me, and I kept wondering what had become of my life. A year ago I was expecting to be married and settled down, and today I was in a dirty cell with twenty sleazy streetwalkers.

"Leave her alone," Georgette said. "She's new to this." And about that time they called us into the courtroom.

There in the audience was Carter, my banker date—sober now—who had been considerate enough to come down to learn what was happening.

Then the lawyer Georgette had engaged for us, who was a relative of the judge, stood up and said his piece. I didn't understand the proceedings too well, but he must have been very competent, because I heard the judge say "Case dismissed."

We all went downstairs for a milkshake and a sandwich, and met the lawyer and Carter. I thanked them both, and I engaged Carter as my banker, which he is to this day.

Then I went uptown to collect my torn addresses from Georgette's laundry, and on to my house, where I drew the curtains and slept for fifteen hours to forget what had been one of the worst nights of my life.

Eight

Puerto Rico

It was February, and New York was bitter cold and buried in slush. I was in no mood to work. The arrest was still on my mind and had left me feeling low.

I was fed up with the whole business of johns, madams, and cops, and the professional environment in general.

I was also lonely, to tell you the truth, because I had split with my last boyfriend, Paul Lindfeld, and everybody else I knew was off to Puerto Rico for Washington's Birthday. I needed to hang loose, breathe free, get lost, take a trip. To hell with it, I'd go to Puerto Rico, too.

I'd never been there before, so I called Pan Am, and they could squeeze me on a flight that was leaving J.F.K. in two hours if I could make it. I didn't even bother to pack properly. I put on a summer dress under my winter coat and stuffed a few essentials in my hand luggage: toothbrush, face creams, diaphragm, and vibrator. I could easily buy whatever else I needed there.

There was enough cash in the house for a round-trip ticket, with $300 left for three days, which was all I expected to stay—at the time.

I paid for my ticket at the airport, and the minute the plane took off I felt better. I looked forward to having some groovy experiences, because I mix easily and have no trouble communicating with people. I believe that's one of the reasons I don't need to drink or smoke cigarettes or grass—I get naturally high on good company.

I was looking forward to a weekend of fun. Work, thank God, was the farthest thing from my mind.

It was hot when we landed in San Juan, people were suntanned, and everything looked sensational. I took a taxi from the airport to the Racquet Club, where some friends were staying, and tried to get a room.

"Forget it, miss," the clerk said. "We can't even rent you a phone booth." This was one of their biggest weekends. So I located my friends, and they invited me to sleep over on their sofa, which was cramped and slightly uncomfortable, but what the hell, it was for a few days only.

Next day I bought a dress, some sandals, and a bikini at the boutique and arranged myself near the pool. The place was overrun with pretty people, mostly couples.

Still, I had a lot of fun meeting people, swimming, sunbathing, and joining the crowd in the afternoons at Fiddler's Green bar for piña coladas, gossip, and dinner arrangements.

For the entire three days, the pattern was pleasant, but so far I had not met anyone who turned me on, and the hot sun was making me hornier than usual. I realized we were near the Virgin Islands, but this celibacy was ridiculous.

On the last afternoon, I met a man named Harry Curtis, a nice blond man from New Hampshire, who had just got off the plane and planned to spend a whole week in Puerto Rico.

He was tall, attractive, intelligent, sensitive, and charming, and after we talked and walked for a while, he invited me to have dinner with him.

That night he took me to romantic Old San Juan, where we ate a delicious paella, walked through the narrow cobblestoned streets, and stopped in a quaint little bar to listen to flamenco guitar music. Then Harry took me home to his room in Carmen's Guest House, and we made marvelous love, after which he suggested I move into his room and spend the next week with him.

That night I brought my things from the Racquet Club to Carmen's cozy guest house and fell madly in love with Harry, forgetting all about returning to New York.

The next week was beautiful. We rented a Volkswagen and drove all over the island together. We made love whenever and wherever we could. On isolated beaches, in the woods, under trees, everywhere.

Harry's cock was tremendous and constantly pulsing with desire. We would make love three and four times in a row, and I would want to do for him things I won't do for every man. I would eat him and swallow his sperm all the way, and I even wanted to have him Greek style, except he was simply too large for that.

After lovemaking we would always talk and laugh and really feel we were in love. It's the most beautiful thing there is, and it's a pity it never lasts forever. When you're fantastically happy, time passes too quickly. Suddenly it was Monday again, and Harry had to leave.

It was time for me to go back also, because it had now been ten days since I impulsively set out for a long weekend, but I wasn't ready to leave. I liked it in San Juan, I felt good, and I looked good. I was as brown as a walnut, my hair was streaked gold from the sun, and I was enjoying my life for the first time in months.

Why should I exchange the sea and the sun in San Juan for the cold and the hassle of New York? I could work just as easily here. I was lucky that I was in a profession that allows me employment no matter where I am.

Although I had been straight since I'd been in Puerto Rico, I had noticed all the potential business hanging around the casinos, the beaches, and the bars.

There was only one obstacle. I had never approached a man on my own before, having always worked through a madam, but I figured there couldn't be anything too difficult about putting together a good sales pitch.

That's one thing I can do well, actually. No matter what business I've been in, I've always been a good saleswoman and actress.

So I sadly said good-bye to Harry, and before he went he paid another week's rent for me at the guest house. We made plans to meet again in New York. He called me twice, but somehow we never did get together.

That morning I got into my bikini and went over to the beach in front of the Americana Hotel to relax and think about my plans. I would have liked to leave a respectable amount of time between seeing my lover off and getting down to business, but I had to be practical because I was down to my last few dollars.

I was tossing up whether I should try to make some money that night, when luck came my way out of the clear blue sky.

It was Mr. Schwartz, sitting not twenty yards away from me, sunning himself with Mrs. Schwartz. I could tell it was Mrs. Schwartz because they looked identical, the way two people do when they have lived together one hundred years.

I recognized him immediately, much to his distress, and when he saw me striding toward him he turned purple. Three weeks before, in New York, Mr. Schwartz had stiffed me for $150 with a bounced check, and when I tried to call him up, the telephone number was a phony. It was divine justice that I ran into him now. But as I approached the couple, the craziest thing happened.

Mr. Schwartz, who was about five years younger than God, whispered something hurriedly to Mrs. Schwartz, who is his approximate contemporary, and they both got up and started to jog!

They both look like they can hardly cross a road in a high wind, and here they were dashing down a beach in the blazing sun. I started to follow, but then I said, To hell with it; he's staying at the Americana, so he has to come back this way if he doesn't drop dead in the meantime.

Now, there is one thing I would rather not do, and that is to embarrass a man in front of his wife. I would never be indiscreet. But if someone deliberately cheats me, then I have no scruples. So I just stood there biding my time, and eventually Mr. Schwartz returned, flushed and puffing, and he looked like a toad.

"Mr. Toad, uh, Mr. Schwartz?" I said, and stepped casually in front of him. He couldn't find his voice and wished he were invisible.

"Aren't you Mr. Schwartz?"

He nodded his head as if to say "Yeah" and got rid of Mrs. Schwartz with the same whispering expertise he used to make her jog down the beach. She was obviously curious, but I'm sure she didn't suspect I was a hooker, because I don't look like one at all.

"Mr. Schwartz," I said, "I would appreciate it if you would give me cash money within the next fifteen minutes, because your check bounced on me.

"If not, it will be the easiest thing in the world to check your room number and tell your wife who I am and what you have done with me.

"Plus, I suggest you should not give phony checks or telephone numbers to girls anymore."

He hurried away and came right back with my $150, and I feel sure it will be a long time before he visits a brothel without something more than his cock in his hand.

So, you see, sometimes a man is forced to be honest by accident. I have been cheated out of so much money it's unbelievable, but that is another story in another chapter.

The next night I made my first professional appearance in the casino to scoop up some of that big bread, but first there were a few things I had to learn about hustling in a place like that.

The first rule to observe is never be too obvious in what you're doing. With big money like that at stake, the house doesn't want some little hustler taking away a high roller who is on either a winning or a losing streak.

If he's winning big, the house will object because they want the chance to win some back.

If he's losing and you say to him "Why continue to lose money on the table, come with me and have some fun," they also react, because you're taking away potential revenue. So either way you have to be cool.

The second rule is don't interrupt a man when he is on a roll. He is likely to be brusque and ask you to go away. Gamblers are known to be very superstitious.

Wait until he is definitely through, and then go in.

I made some mistakes, understandably, on the first night, but after that I quickly learned how to operate. To begin with, I walked in wearing one of those see-through dresses, very transparent, very sexy and revealing, and the whole room noticed me and went *grrrrowl*.

The women, most of all, said, "Look at that girl, she has nothing underneath, not even underpants!"

Next thing I knew I was taken out like a little pussycat: "Lady, would you please remove yourself from the premises?" Carlos, the pit boss, said.

I didn't know they were so strict in their rules of dress. Squares! So I made it with Carlos, and that saved my head, but he warned me: "Xaviera, please try not to be so conspicuous in the future."

I came back again fully dressed, wearing no makeup—just a little eye shadow and lip gloss—and making, I believe, a clean, fresh impression. I also behaved conservatively, but by now the men were watching me like wolves.

I picked out a man who was playing with $100 and $50 chips who had no woman beside him, and he was my target. I stood back, caught his eye, gave him a suggestive smile and a sexy look, and he noticed me.

Then I worked my way in beside him, and at the first opportunity, asked him to teach me a few gambling rules.

"Wait just a while," he said, "and we'll go have a drink at the bar, and I'll explain them to you."

When he was through, we went to the bar, chatted a while, and I said, "I guess you're here with your wife?"

"No, I'm here alone," he said, "so why don't we go up to my room and discuss the rules of gambling?"

In the first week or two, I took my prospects to the bar and gave them a little sales talk, changing it each day to add something nice and personal about each man. I usually gave them the story that I was a secretary from the United Nations in Puerto

Rico on vacation and trying to earn just $50 to pay for my hotel room. Telling a man that kind of story makes him feel he is not dealing with a prostitute.

However, if the man asked me to stay over in his room for the night, I said, "I would love to, but you will definitely have to raise the fee to $150."

But I never asked for cash up front, because that strikes me as too whorish.

As my action accelerated, I dropped the bar and the corny story about the rules of gambling or being a secretary on vacation, because it was all too time-consuming. Instead I developed a smooth, nonchalant way of shopping the men with an arrogant look and a subtle shake of the head—left to right, yes or no—and we got straight down to business. Most men are happy to do that and get back to the tables, and pretty soon I was well established, making $200 to $300 a day, plus I had tons of time left to relax on the beach and do my own private thing.

My daily routine usually was as follows: In the morning I went to the beach, found a canvas chair, sunbathed, swam, and fooled around with some young kid.

One of my favorite pastimes still is to seduce young, innocent boys of about seventeen. My technique is to make friends with their parents, and while I chat them up, start discreetly flirting with sonny boy. That year, my luck was in; everybody seemed to have taken their sons on vacation to Puerto Rico. So, during the conversation, I would suggest that the young man might like to have a walk along the beach. Once we found a deserted spot, we would go for a swim, preferably naked, and that would be followed by a bout of "fooling around." There was always the possibility of being discovered, so for a favored few, I would take them back to my room and give them "the works."

Young boys, with their rock-hard cocks, would generally come within seconds, and I would persevere to teach them how to control themselves and avoid premature ejaculation. In fact, I would treat them to a complete course on how to be nice and unselfish and what to do and where to do it, their education being completed with an oral test. They were so eager to learn and grateful—without any trace of conceit—and they were never blasé.

So, late in the afternoon, I would send these boys who had suddenly become *men* back to their unsuspecting parents. Or maybe Momma or Poppa did wonder why junior should flop back in such an exhausted state onto his beach blanket after a leisurely walk along the seashore.

If I may be immodest for a minute, I will estimate that 25 percent of all Jewish youths who vacationed in Puerto Rico between February and April 1970 were taught the art of love by me. A few fathers, customers who thought I was just a horny college girl paying her way with favors, even chipped in and paid me to educate their sons.

Around 4:00 P.M., when the sun was no longer strong, and the bars were closing for siesta, I would set out to turn two tricks. My daytime working area was around the lobby of the Americana or the El San Juan Hotel, where I would stand outside the bar or the drugstore and approach a likely looking customer on the spot.

If the man's wife was out shopping or getting her hair done, we would go up to his room, and I would blow him, fuck him, boom, boom, fifteen minutes, $50, and out.

If their wives were around, they would usually give me their card and say: "I can't do anything here, but call me in New York."

Occasionally I would hand them my card, but as a rule that is a dangerous practice, because their wives could discover it in their pockets. In New York, card passing is acceptable because prostitutes disguise their profession by printing on them activities like objets d'art, management consultants, or, in my case, interior designer. However, others are more obvious, and if a sharp wife finds a card in her husband's pocket with one of the following occupations—headmistress, erection and demolition expert, public relations, or even manual laborer—she can usually assume the only thing getting made is himself.

After two customers, I would go back to the guest house, take a siesta until around 10:00 P.M., bathe, dress, and have a bite to eat at the Lemon Tree in the El San Juan before setting out for my night's work. My target was four customers a day—two in the afternoon and two at night—because I wanted some time to myself, and frankly, could not easily handle any more on my own.

However, I was obliged to make an exception in certain cases. There was the time the group of eight New Jersey Italians vacationed in San Juan for a week, and all kept wanting to get laid at once.

They would send their wives out shopping around ten in the morning and take me to their cabana at the Americana and screw me one by one while somebody watched the door to make sure the women did not return and catch them.

They would be joking and turning on to the outrageousness of the scene as much as to getting laid.

Once this same horny group arranged to meet me on the beach at midnight while their wives were all occupied at the tables playing roulette or blackjack.

It was a beautiful, idyllic setting under the stars with a warm breeze blowing and the waves gently crashing in the background, but the lovemaking was far from romantic.

As they stood in line laughing and unzipping their pants, I

gave them each a blow job on the sand. I was blowing and spitting and blowing again and wishing I had my bottle of mouthwash with me, or at least a water fountain to rinse my mouth out, because the taste of so much sperm really turns me off, and that night it almost made me vomit.

I am used to a more sophisticated way of operating, but these guys didn't care about white sheets, only about getting their rocks off before their wives discovered they were missing.

I was not wearing any panties while I was kneeling down on the beach blowing them, and the mosquitoes started biting my bare bottom. Then the guard dog from the hotel came barking around, followed by the night watchman, who threw a flashlight beam on us and ran away, shocked.

Altogether, it was a complicated and uncomfortable way of conducting business on both sides, so I settled for a ten-dollar reduction per man on a package deal for a group of eight.

Business was booming, and I was making a fortune, but Carmen's Guest House was becoming an inconvenient place to stay. Apart from the fact that it was too far removed from the action, I suspected they were starting to figure out just what my activity was, and in a little place like that, word soon gets around. So I started thinking about moving out of there.

A few days later I met a young man on the beach named David, who was around twenty-eight, much older than my usual freebie. He approached me, and asked me would I like to go for a row on his rubber raft.

The funny thing was that on that day I had an invitation to go sailing on a huge luxury yacht, but David's suggestion appealed to me more.

We paddled a long way out to sea, talking and laughing and falling into the water and scrambling back on board, and as I hung on to his strong, sunburned shoulders, I started to get really turned on.

He wasn't good-looking, but he had a sexy, rugged, Jean-Paul Belmondo kind of face, and he also had a big Jewish nose. There's a saying in German—*"An dem Nasen eines Mannes erkennt man sein Johannes"*—which means you can guess the size of a man's penis by the size of his nose.

I also believe you can tell from his hands. If he has long, slim fingers, he usually has a long, slim cock. If he has short, thick fingers, he usually has a short, thick cock, and if he has meaty, fleshy hands like a butcher, he usually has a flabby, fleshy cock.

I take the liberty of making these generalizations because I have done enough penetrating research in my time to consider myself an expert on the subject.

After paddling around for a while, David and I came back ashore, left the raft in the shade to dry out, and went to the hotel's outdoor bar for a piña colado and a fruit punch, my favorite drink. There we met his roommates, Ricky, Hood, and Brian, and together we spent the rest of the afternoon running around the beach, talking, and, of course, getting around to the topic of sex.

The boys, aged between twenty-eight and thirty-two, complained how square the vacationing New York girls were and how innocent and stupid. "What we need for us is a woman like you," David said, to which the others all agreed. When one of them suggested I move into their guest house, I jumped at the idea.

Why not? Their place was close by the beach and the action, and what more could I want than four strong, horny young men to play with in my free time?

We all walked over to the little white two-story clapboard house, where we found the landlady, a dear old German grandmother type, in the garden watering her plants.

I approached her in German requesting a room, and she was so charmed and flattered that she said I could have the best room, on the boys' floor, with air-conditioning and a bathroom all to myself. The guest house was modest but clean and unbelievably cheap for Puerto Rico: only $10 a day.

"Okay, I'll move in," I told the boys. "So let's go over to Carmen's and get my belongings."

When the boys brought me back with my luggage, which had increased since I arrived in Puerto Rico, they went to their own room to freshen up and relax, and I went to mine down the hall to unpack.

Half an hour later I went to their room, which was very big and had several single beds in it, and I found them all fresh out of the shower with towels around them—all except David, who was walking around naked, and proving my theory about big noses.

There was the smell of grass in the room, and they were lazily smoking, and the sound of rock music was roaring in the background. Soon somebody suggested we have an orgy to celebrate my arrival.

Nobody needed much persuasion, and pretty soon we were all stripped naked, tangled on the floor between the beds, sucking, fucking, blowing, laughing, and climaxing. It was an unbelievably beautiful scene. Our bodies were hot and perspiring because there was no air-conditioning in their room, so we showered and did it all again.

Caught up in the abandon of the whole scene, I forgot my resolution never to allow compromising photos to be taken of me.

We took out the Polaroid camera to make some pictures, one of which was an absolute masterpiece. The tourist bureau should have used it on a postcard. It was a picture of me wearing David's Spanish matador hat, sitting on his cock on the floor, while Ricky was standing on my right getting a blow job and Brian to my left getting a hand job.

Hood, the one who took the pictures, had never been in a group scene before, and he was so bashful he could not get it up, so I had to fuck him privately in my room later on.

As we jumped around and carried on, I started to get a sneaking feeling that somehow we were being watched. Nobody else seemed to notice, but they were so whacked out of their heads on grass that they couldn't care less if we were on *Candid Camera*.

But I couldn't shake the feeling there was someone observing our scene, and as I looked toward the window that led onto the veranda, I saw the venetian-blind slats move almost imperceptibly.

Without being obvious and not saying a word, I casually climbed off David's cock and walked to the bureau under the window, pretending to get something in a drawer.

When my hand was out of eye range, I took hold of the blind cord and yanked it open, and there, staring me in the face, were the startled eyes of the landlady's forty-five-year-old spinster daughter. Her peroxide-blond hair was all matted in the perspiration on her forehead. She was blushing and was very embarrassed indeed.

"Madam," I said to her, "would you please keep your nose out of private parties unless you are invited? Furthermore, I would be grateful if you do not shock the sweet old landlady by telling her what you have seen."

Without saying a word, she hurried away along the veranda, and we all cracked up laughing. And that, more or less, was the reckless tone of my next few weeks with the band of vagabonds.

The boys were on "extended" vacation in Puerto Rico, living the best way they could, which was not always something their parents would approve of if they knew. They were all law-school graduates, except David, the dropout, who was a larcenist by nature and the biggest, horniest fuck of all.

But Hood was the one I liked best emotionally. He was sensitive, intelligent, and from an aristocratic New Jersey family. Together we all lived like beach bums, wildly and sometimes childishly, but it was a good balance for the work I was doing twice daily.

In the mornings we would all go to the beach, pinch some chairs, fool around, then around 4:00 P.M. I would leave for my afternoon's business and join the boys back at the house later for a mini-orgy and a siesta.

If the landlady's nosy daughter was still interested in our activities, she no longer showed it, and always made a point of darting out of sight whenever my band of "freak hippies" walked by.

However, one morning when I broke our regular routine by being absent from the house all day and ducked back to pick up my suntan lotion, I discovered that I was wrong.

As I climbed the wooden stairs, I could see the sandaled feet of the spinster daughter standing motionless beside my bed. Oh, my God, I thought, the busybody old snoop has found our orgy pictures. Then I remembered she had seen the live performance, so what the hell, let her have her kicks as long as the dear old landlady was not exposed to it.

But as I tiptoed barefoot into the room, I saw none other than the old lady herself holding our pictures up to the light and discussing our various positions as though she and her daughter were Masters and Johnson!

They were both so absorbed in the pornography that they didn't hear me enter at first.

"Good morning, ladies," I said. "Are you enjoying our happy snaps?"

They wheeled around, mouths open, dropped the pictures like hot coals into the open drawer, and slammed it shut.

"Madam," I addressed myself to the daughter, "it is not enough that you snoop around things that don't concern you, but you have to get an innocent old lady involved too. You should be ashamed of yourself, you really should."

They didn't wait to hear any more, they just bowed their heads and hurried straight out of the room.

I was angry in a way, but at the same time grateful that the pictures were the only thing they found—because stashed away in my pocketbooks, luggage lining, and even my passport were bundles of fifties, twenties, and tens, which represented most of my three months' earnings.

One night I met in the casino a likable man in his forties named Larry Dreyfus. He was tall and handsome, with silver-gray hair, and he was kind and attentive. He took me to dinner and taught me to gamble, so that I soon preferred shooting craps to turning tricks. Larry was an insurance adjuster in New York, and when the time came for him to leave, I trusted him sufficiently to give him an envelope in which I had placed a few thousand dollars to keep safe for me until I managed to get back to the Big Apple. Opening a bank account in Puerto Rico would have been a complicated business. I did not think it wise to leave money lying about where any nosy landlady might find it, and I had my doubts about the honesty of my playmates, such as David.

To show you what David was like, in the nighttime we would all get dressed up, and he would take us to the most expensive restaurants in San Juan in a hot VW and pay for the multicourse banquets with stolen credit cards. If he could do something straight, he would reject it, because he got a great deal of genuine pleasure out of being crooked. There was nothing he loved to do more than give his friends a good time on other people's money.

As the weeks went on, our behavior became more and more reckless and abandoned, and we would do almost anything that had an air of danger about it, which is why one day David suggested we all get stoned on mescaline.

As I mentioned, I don't use stimulants of any sort, not even coffee, so at first I was naturally scared. But David assured me everything would be all right, especially as we would all take a pill each together, and the effects would last no longer than eight or nine hours.

David knew all about drugs—as well as turning on to them, he also pushed them on occasional trips to Miami—so we took his word for it.

It was a Friday morning when we went on our "trip." We took the yellow capsules around noon as we left the guest house and in a "temporarily borrowed" Volkswagen drove to a small secluded beach ten minutes from San Juan.

By the time we arrived, the stuff was beginning to work. It was a perfect spot; the long beach of white sand was completely deserted, a veritable paradise. We piled out of the car, and all our inhibitions were blown away in the breeze. Even the retiring Hood came out of his shell, and we tore off our clothes and plunged into the sea. Soon we were playing games, singing songs, and making love—in fact, doing anything that came into our heads, reveling in our total freedom. Somebody tried to take some Polaroids but, after a couple of bungled attempts, dropped the camera into the water. I badly needed a pee, which is not something that I would normally do in public, unless it was part of a freak scene for which I was going to be paid. Now, however, I was so abandoned that I shouted to everybody a report on the state of my bladder, spread my legs wide, threw my ass in the air, and let go. Then I felt David's cock rammed hard against my pissing pussy. I was still peeing when he shot his load against my clitoris. The others were in a frenzy, thrashing about in the sand or jerking off in front of me. The whole scene was like a speeded-up movie of ourselves, which we were watching from somewhere outside.

Colors became very vibrant. The sun was like a golden ball dangling above our heads, and the sea was like blue Jell-O oozing to shore and out again. We ran into the hills and made love with a background of palm trees threaded by a sandy road that we must have come along, which appeared to lead into a small village.

As we were tripping out and jumping around, a maroon car passed on the road, looking as if it were from a different world, but somehow very close, and inside was a Negro who looked out, waved, and drove on.

You don't entirely lose your head on mescaline, and even though you're stoned, you still know what's happening. Pretty soon the same maroon car was back again, this time carrying three Negroes, all waving. Then it went away again.

Five minutes later, or an hour—we could not judge time any-more—the same car came along followed by a sight-seeing bus full of blacks staring at those nude people jumping around out there.

The bus slowed, stopped, then took off again, but the three blacks parked the maroon car near the palm trees and started wading through the water to us. As they got closer, I got this obsession that I wanted to see them jerking off. I had never made love with a black man, but I had heard the story that they are all huge. So I indicated my desire by making the manual gesture, up and down, and indeed one of them took out his cock and started jerking off! Then the others started doing it, too.

Just then a bunch of schoolkids with their satchels on their backs appeared. The Negroes retreated into the bushes while we were still doing our thing, and the children were walking backward, looking at us with eyes like saucers.

From beneath the palm trees the blacks were trying to hit me with coconuts, and at this point we started to realize we should split. But now we were so stoned we could not control anything anymore.

"Xaviera, get dressed, put your clothes on," one of the boys said. So I grabbed my bikini underpants and tied them around my neck, which was my way of covering up in front of the kids and the blacks.

We tried to gather up our belongings from the sand, but for some reason our fingers were insensitive, and we could not hold them. Combs, lipsticks, wallets, and suntan oil dropped from our hands. We left them in the sand and ran to the VW.

Nobody was really capable of driving, but Ricky took the wheel, and we zigzagged back to San Juan, almost hitting a tree and a boy on a bicycle, and came to a stop inside the garden of the El San Juan Hotel.

It was the cocktail hour, nearly dusk, and as we jumped from the car all the Jewish American Princesses moved away from us with the look of, "Oh, boy, look at those animals." I took one look at myself in a car mirror, with my eyes like red Frisbees, made a dash to the water, and paddled out to sea on David's raft.

By around nine that night the mescaline had almost worn off, but we hadn't been home to change, so I went to work just as I was, wearing pigtails and my bikini bottoms and a little beach dress, slightly high and giggling.

I looked more like a crazy beach virgin than a hooker, and I turned on quite a few older men, who paid a fortune, and it was my biggest night apart from the Mafia blow jobs.

As Easter approached, three months after I arrived for three days in Puerto Rico, I started getting bored. Among other things, all the boys had gone home, except David, who was down on his luck and depended on me for ten- and twenty-dollar handouts every now and again. I even let him live in my room, as I had more or less moved into a gorgeous penthouse with a gambler named Norris, who wasn't a john and would not pay me, but let me have anything I needed in the way of clothes or food.

Two days before Easter David said he was going to Miami on a dope deal to make a lot of money and would be away for a week, leaving at six o'clock in the evening.

After the other boys left, David and I had an intense kind of platonic friendship, so I wanted to get back from the beach early and say good-bye and perhaps go with him to the airport. But as I returned from the beach around four o'clock, I could sense something was wrong. All was quiet in my room, and as I walked in the door I was horrified to find it looked like a tornado had hit it.

Drawers and dresses were inside out, clothes were all over the place, my luggage was lying open in the room, and the lining had been ripped open and the money stolen.

I ran to my closet and plunged my hand into every pocket on every dress I had, and they were all empty. Even my pocketbook had been cleaned out, and the notes stuffed into my passport were also missing.

Whoever did it really cleaned me out. There was enough to make one phone call: two nickels.

I had to find David. He was due to leave in a couple of hours, but if I could get him first, he might be able to help me out, because he knew every thief in Puerto Rico.

I ran down to the beach where Beegee, his little hippie girlfriend, hung around pushing grass. "Have you seen David around?" I asked her.

"I sure did," she said. "About an hour ago, on his way to the airport."

"On his way to the airport?" I said. "Are you sure? He's not leaving for two hours."

"That's not what he told me," Beegee said. "He was dashing to the airport carrying his bag, and he asked me to mind it and his suede coat while he went into the hotel to make a phone call.

"Come to think of it, he was very nervous about the coat and said don't let anybody get their hands on it, and the pockets and lining seemed to be stuffed with paper."

I got the message loud and clear. My friend David, whom I had virtually supported for the last few weeks, had done the robbery. So much for honor among thieves.

I ran to the roadway, flagged down a cruising police car, and managed to talk them into taking me to San Juan Airport to try to catch him.

I knew he had hot tickets under the name of L. Lieberman, and as far as I knew, takeoff time was an hour away.

At the airport I went straight to the departure counter to check out the flight. There was no Lieberman on the 6:00 P.M. flight, the clerk told me, but Mr. L. Lieberman was on board the plane just taking off. There was no way of stopping him, so I was wiped out, ripped off, $3,000 gone. I could only take a philosophical look at the situation and say easy come, easy go, and just as well. I still had my round-trip ticket and *mens sana in corpore sano*—sound mind in sound body.

Nine

Call Me Madam

For two months after returning from Puerto Rico, I operated as an independent call girl, or *loner,* as they are known, until it struck me that this was an unsatisfactory way to earn a living.

Loners make a maximum of $300 from an average of four customers a night, and their income depends on pleasing a loyal but limited clientele that does not demand too much in the way of variety.

However, in order to give a client an occasional change of face, they form into tight little groups and exchange dates among themselves. For example, Gloria will send a customer to Sandy, who will send one back to her. But if Sandy cannot reciprocate, she must pay Gloria a madam's fee of usually 40 percent of what the client paid her.

Working this way, the girls protect themselves to a certain extent from the competition, but it's only a matter of time before some pretty, young newcomer squeezes into the circle and seduces away their business.

I recognized this john-swapping activity as bringing in a lot of new faces but no extra money, and that in the end, loners could only be losers. More to the point, I believed I had the qualities it takes to be a successful madam: aggressive leadership, a head for figures, a love of people, and matchless stamina. I can get by on four or five hours' sleep a night for an entire year if necessary.

But above all I had what I call the "madam instinct": the ability to know when to be bitchy or soft, the diplomacy to handle difficult clients, good hostess skills, and above all, a sense of humor.

And ever since I left the straight life behind, I'd wanted to make it big in this business. So in the summer of 1970 I decided to become not just a madam—but the best in New York.

The first thing I had to do was to find a good location to open up shop. Working as a loner is one thing, and it's a rare Manhattan building that does not have at least one discreet house hooker, but finding a place to open a lively brothel was a different story.

The ideal building, first of all, has to have the proper climate: cool. This means that the management and staff will tolerate, cooperate, and even protect you as long as you cross their palms with silver.

However, this can go too far, and there is one luxury high-rise in the East Fifties with such an army of cooperative doormen and lobby staff that it was costing Georgette Harcourte almost $500 each month, before rent, when she operated there.

There are several buildings on Manhattan's smart East Side that are known to tolerate active brothels. One harbors so many it is called the Vertical Whorehouse. This building, located on York Avenue in the Seventies, advertises in the real-estate columns of the *New York Times* as having "the ultimate in services and conveniences." Another building riddled with brothels is on Sutton Place, but as far as I could see, these addresses were no longer cool—they were red hot, with the police watching them like hawks.

It took some searching, but eventually I found the perfect place: a one-bedroom apartment in the East Fifties on a commercial floor of a semicommercial building—which meant there would be no neighbors to worry about after office hours. Initially I wanted a modest apartment that would keep my overhead down. I knew that I could utilize the living room as well as the bedroom for entertaining my customers.

The next step was to recruit staff, and believe it or not, honest, hardworking hookers are hard to find. There were girls around who worked the cheap houses, but they were mostly hardened creatures, and I would not then, nor will I now, ever use a girl who has no class. I don't want street hookers, because their mentality is too cheap. I have a classy clientele who pay high prices for class. If a man would never pick up a girl in the street, why should I expect him to go with a street hooker?

At one point I hired a girl who had worked in a cheap house, and as a result, got exactly what I should have expected: cheap behavior. In this case I relaxed my policy because the girl, Misty, was outwardly attractive. But when she undressed, there were stretch marks all over her body from children she gave birth to when she was fourteen and fifteen. At nineteen, when she came to me, she was already used up. And I soon found out her niceness was a very thin veneer.

As is my practice with new girls, I gave Misty a pleasant, attractive man as her first customer. The man, a stockbroker, was slightly drunk but the easy-to-handle type.

Misty retired to the bedroom with him, but within five minutes dramatically reappeared, charging stark naked into the living room, cursing and swearing.

So I went inside and walked into a screaming match between the customer and Misty. "Listen," I cried, taking the customer's side, "you're not working in a twenty-five-dollar whorehouse, so don't behave like a whore!"

"Goddamnit!" she screamed. "I've already taken care of that bastard, and now he wants some more!"

It is my philosophy that a man is entitled to more than five minutes of a girl's time, and even if he climaxes quickly, he can expect to be treated warmly and even babied and washed up if that's what he wants.

Misty quieted down and promised to cooperate, but her background was too strong, and twice a day I had complaints that she was a hard, cold bitch. So I had to dismiss her.

The others who were not attached to madams already usually had a pimp behind the scenes and pimps are bad news, because sooner or later they try to move in on your business.

In the beginning I did hire some girls who had pimps, and only one of them, a lovely looking blonde named Leonora, worked out well. I met Leonora through a fifty-year-old pimp named Tony Roland, who was known to handle the best-looking "working" girls in New York, and he saw that they were punctual and reliable. However, this particular girl had aspirations higher than hooking, and through a customer of mine, landed herself a television commercial, and her face is now splashed across the home screen.

The exceptional thing about this story is not that a prostitute achieved legitimate fame, because some major celebrities we all know began that way, but that her pimp let her get out of the business. But I suppose she is making more money now as a minor celebrity, and in this way, Tony is still her old man.

An unhappy case of one pimp refusing to let go of his bread-and-butter body was Greta, a small-time madam who operated from the York Avenue building. She was managed by a "connected" Italian who took care of payoffs and made sure she never got busted. But the pimp himself got sent away for armed robbery. This did not make him surrender his suffocating hold on the girl; even from prison he managed her via two of his lieutenants, who kept her under twenty-four-hour surveillance—even when she went out to visit her mother in Queens.

Different madams have different methods of finding girls to work for them, and on a couple of occasions I tried to follow their examples.

A lesbian madam named Janet cruises the gay-girl bars like Cookies, The Tree, and Harry's Back East to find working girls. She finds some little dyke, seduces her, invites her to live in her apartment for a few days, then persuades her to go into the game. This isn't too difficult with lesbians, because basically they hate men and enjoy taking their money in exchange for sex.

I tried Janet's approach one night in Maxwell's Plum. I struck up a conversation with a gorgeous, straight, gray-eyed girl in the powder room.

"You're a very lovely looking girl," I said. "Are you by any chance a model?"

The girl stopped applying her lipstick. "Oh, no, I'm just a secretary," she said.

"How come you dress so beautifully on a secretary's salary?" I asked. "Do you have a rich fiancé?"

"Heavens, no," she laughed. "I wish I did, then I wouldn't have to spend every cent I earn on clothes."

"A girl like you should not have to work; you should have men spending money on you," I told her. She was so delicious, I would have liked to make love to her myself.

"Where can I find that?" she asked, showing casual but genuine interest.

"I know lots of rich men who would like to spoil you. Are you interested?"

"Oh, sure, I'm interested," she said earnestly. "As long as there's no sex involved."

I met a cute girl named Jenny at a gay bar, and although my intention was not exactly recruitment, it developed that way.

Jenny was twenty but looked fourteen, with short gamin hair, and she told me she had never had sex with anyone but was butch.

"It's impossible to be butch when you are a virgin," I explained. "You become one gradually after having sex. You might look a little tomboyish with your short hair, but to me, you're feminine—so let me be the butch."

Jenny had a beautiful body, with thick, black pubic hair, and she turned me on tremendously. However, she wasn't clean and fresh down there, and I had to teach her all about hygiene and how to wash up, because she couldn't douche, being a virgin, with her hymen still in place.

We'd sit in a tub together, and I would play with her little titties and suck them and go down on her. I adored her so much I became protective toward her, like a lover. I adored the way she kissed me with her full, sensual mouth.

Poor little Jenny was slightly chaotic in her private life. She couldn't keep a job; she was always broke, and at one point didn't even have a place to stay. I let her move in with me for a while, but it was no atmosphere for a virgin. So I decided she had to get enough money to take care of herself, and I suggested earning it from my customers.

"Look," I said, "I've got a couple of johns coming up tonight. You can earn a quick fifty, and you don't have to fuck, just blow."

She'd never given a blow job; in fact, she had never seen a cock in her life, so I taught her on a banana, and she seemed, timidly, to get the hang of it.

That night when the two customers came up, I had decided to entertain them in the bathtub, because some men love to watch girls performing their ablutions, among other things, especially if one of them is like a little baby. But these two horny bastards got so excited seeing us in the bath, they took off their pants immediately and stuck their cocks into our mouths. All of a sudden I felt afraid for Jenny. At least these guys were circumcised, but hers got very carried away and was being very rough.

Jenny was holding on to me like a little kitten, and she was making choking sounds, and her neck was convulsing because he was penetrating too far. She was definitely not ready for deep-throating. Then this bastard came down her throat, and the poor little mouse vomited and started to cry. Clearly, sweet little Jenny was not cut out for this calling.

Somehow, short of advertising in the *New York Times*, I felt there had to be a source of enthusiastic amateurs who could be turned into gifted professionals. Quite by accident I came upon a virtual De Beers diamond field of untapped talent when a friend named Norman took me one late-summer weekend to a nudist camp.

This was my first experience with en masse nudism, and although I certainly was not inhibited, it was a case of not quite knowing where to put one's hands, figuratively as well as literally. However, it wasn't long before I was given my direction.

As I sat by the edge of the pool, just taking in the scene, my eyes fell on a rather enchanting sight. Sitting a few yards away from me, in the middle of a group of people, was a woman with stunning red hair and a silky pubic triangle to match. As I watched, this inviting flame sparkled at me, and she moved her legs so that I could have a closer look, almost inside her vagina. And I must say that had I been a man my anatomy would have betrayed my mentality. As I wondered what to do next, I caught sight of the suntanned lifeguard, who had been watching the silent exchange and now gave me a wink and a beckoning look.

I walked over to where he sat, and before I spoke he said, "I can tell you how to join in with that interesting group if you want to."

"I'd like very much to meet them," I said.

"Very well," he said, "they are a sort of a club, and all you need is the right introductory passwords."

"They call themselves Tulips, and they are French, so give it a try."

I walked straight over to the flame's circle and said, "*Bonjour, madame. Je m'appelle Xaviera, moi aussi, je suis une tulipe de la Hollande*." "Good day, Madame. My name is Xaviera, and I also am a tulip from Holland." Little did they know how accurate that was.

A pleasant wave of laughter went through the group, there were introductions all around, and before I could say "Adam and Eve," they invited me for a drink inside their cabana.

Six of us crowded into the small room, which contained two single beds, and little else, and without too much need for formality, I was soon eating my way through my flaming redhead's pussy. She was in her forties, I guessed, but she had a nice firm body, flat stomach, and strong breasts. Her inviting vagina was warm and exciting, and my tongue darted through her curly red hair as I was stretched out between her legs. I licked and sucked her clitoris with my vibrating tongue until it was hard and erect.

Meanwhile, the flame's husband was standing with his face very close to the action to see exactly what it was I was doing to make his wife moan, writhe, and have multiple climaxes. Each time she was exhausted, but I would work her up to a new orgasm with my tongue, which never seemed to tire. She tasted delicious, and my face was wet, and by this time I had made her climax three times.

As I finally stopped eating her, her husband, who had been waiting, all turned on, with a big erection, put his cock into the now soaking-wet vagina of the flame, and it was a pleasure to watch them make love.

Her whole body was perspiring, and the squishy-squashy noises turned everybody else on. Only then did I become aware of all the other people, because I was concentrating only on my flame. But my hunger for pussy was not yet sated, and several other girls who had been turned on and were going crazy at the ecstatic pleasure the flame was enjoying wanted me to suck their pussies too.

Afterward I was exhausted, and the orgy I had started was going strong, but some of the girls and guys went for a swim to freshen up and cool off, and there I ran into my companion, Norman.

"Go inside that cabana," I told him, "and you will have a ball." I didn't see Norman again for another two hours, but while I was sitting around with some of the naked females, I found it easy to convince them that their generous-spirited talents could be

gainfully employed, and some of them agreed to become working girls at my house.

As I expected, these women turned out to be great professionals, because they were uninhibited in their approach, yet
decent types of girls.

One of my first and most successful girls was a stewardess
from El Al airlines, who was very popular until she got rerouted
and we lost her. Stewardesses often drift easily into the professional life as a supplemental income, starting out with having
flings with married men from the first-class cabin, then asking
themselves why do this for free? After awhile, they do regular
stints in houses from Hong Kong to Helsinki, and London to
Los Angeles, in their layover time, of course.

Among my early girls was also a young Englishwoman, a former stewardess, recently separated from her violent American
husband, she just wanted to make enough money to support
herself and pay for her divorce action.

How many times I wished my business were legal so I could,
indeed, advertise in the employment columns of the newspapers: good pay, flexible hours, opportunity to meet lots of men.

Another madam I knew recruited her staff entirely from
among bored Westchester housewives, and her house in
Manhattan flourishes on a modest scale to this day. Inés was a
Cuban woman who married an American, went to live in
Westchester, and spent her days sitting around with other
neglected wives listening to them talk about how they screwed
the window washer, the gardener, the delivery man, and anything moving slower than three miles an hour.

"Listen," she said to them, "if you like sex so much, why
don't you come down to Manhattan with me and make money
out of it?"

Inés herself got divorced and devoted her time to running the brothel in a midtown apartment, and the girls worked for her in rotating shifts. But she had her staff problems, too, because married women are always taking time off to go on vacation with their husbands or to have babies and hysterectomies.

I started hiring girls who had daytime jobs as secretaries and salesgirls and wanted to make some money on the side. I found they were less jaded and more enthusiastic than a working girl who's been screwing her brains out ten times a day in another house. Many successful call girls, on the other hand, are also known to be cold and businesslike.

The girls with whom I carried on a terrific business were usually foreigners who had no work permit but had to support themselves—and sometimes a child. Blondes were in great demand.

The next step was promotion. A high-class house advertises strictly by word of mouth of satisfied customers, and never goes out soliciting.

Other areas of prostitution go to any lengths to solicit business, like the semilegit massage parlors that even put cute girls on Lexington Avenue these days posing as poll-takers. The only answers they want are the man's opinion of "special massage," his name, and office telephone number.

Others, as we all know, openly harass people in the streets, and in hotels, and sometimes even savagely attack them.

An operation like mine never approaches people but waits for the customers to come because they're interested. In other words, it's a supply situation strictly catering to a demand. And as long as there is such a thing as male libido, the ostrich-attitude law notwithstanding, there will always be a demand for a fancy brothel.

For me business opened with a bang, so to speak, because I had a very good reputation in the profession as a quantity-as-well-as-quality girl.

Word spread around, and within a month or two of my opening there was almost too much business to handle in a one-bedroom apartment.

Some nights were so packed that there would be two couples using the king-sized bed at the same time, another couple using the queen-sized Castro convertible in the living room, and yet another pair in the cot set up in the corner.

Still others would be in the kitchen boozing and lining up for their turn; those who were impatient or in a hurry would sometimes settle for a blow job in the bathroom.

By the end of the year, business was so fantastically successful that I had to look for a bigger apartment. I was so happy at the way things were going that I sent out Christmas cards to my clients to let them know I was moving and that I had a "new stable" for them to look over, and the card listed my new phone number.

This move got me into a little hot water when one customer called up and said his wife had received the card and demanded to know who was Madam Xaviera and what was her stable.

"You have to get me out of the hole now," he ranted. "I know she intends calling you up, so you'd better make sure you tell her you are a horse trainer."

The new apartment I found was a three-bedroom place in the East Sixties in an entirely residential building, but with a cooperative door staff.

The week I signed the lease, I had a phone call from my former madam and chief competitor, Madeleine, whom I had not spoken to for almost a year, since she had stopped using me.

Some drunk had left my card lying around, and she found it and I can't blame her for being mad at me.

However, I was not surprised to hear from her now.

Through the infallible grapevine, I knew that she was getting out of the business to get married for the fourth time, and her attempts to put someone in the house on a managerial basis had been disasters.

The first girl she tried was Anita, a sweet young thing who would make a perfect courtesan but who lacked the madam instinct.

The second choice was even more naive. I never thought of Madeleine as a gullible woman, but she really goofed choosing Linda. Linda was a junkie, and the one thing you cannot tolerate in a house is drugs, because if the police find them, you haven't a leg to stand on. Blind Freddie, one of her butlers, could see that the bandages on the girl's hands covered up the needle marks, but for some reason Madeleine didn't.

As well as being a hard-core user, Linda was entirely chaotic in her personal life and had no idea of how to handle finances. But worse than all that, she failed the acid test—to get along with the scheming butler, Felipe. Felipe worked by day in a brokerage house on Wall Street; by night he functioned as a sort of general factotum, taking hats and coats, ferrying girls to and from dates, and arranging payoffs. But I never liked or trusted the man. In my opinion, he had a double tongue as well as a double life, but he had a lot of influence with Madeleine.

Felipe also was a snoop, and one day while poking around Linda's apartment, he found her needles and other equipment and informed Madeleine, who had to let her go.

So here she was calling me up and inviting me over for coffee that same afternoon to discuss a matter "of some extreme urgency."

There was a little sadness in me when I arrived at the elegant brownstone on East Twenty-seventh Street, to realize that one of New York's more exciting institutions was, despite the fact it was a rival establishment, closing down.

Madeleine, immaculate and elegant as usual, answered the door, ushered me into her private sitting room, and without beating about the bush began. "I think you know why I have asked you here," she said in her South African English.

"I have heard some talk about your retiring," I said.

"I just got married, and I am pregnant already. Now you see why I need somebody who is able to take over my operation," she said.

"Why did you call me?" I asked.

"I'll be quite honest and admit that I didn't give you first offer, but after a couple of failures to keep the house operating, I have realized you are the only person in New York who can run it.

"I've watched how you built yourself up from a little secretary who used to do scenes in her lunch hour to become one of the best madams in town in less than a year, and I admire you for it. I think you are ready to take over my business, and the only question now is, do you want it?"

Madeleine's was known to be the biggest business in town. So by acquiring it, I would become New York's reigning madam.

However, I was not interested in Felipe whom I never trusted or the five-story brownstone. I much preferred the relaxed atmosphere of walking from room to room to supervise instead of climbing all those flights of stairs.

"How much do you want for your black book and your tele-phone lines?" I asked.

Madeleine asked for a down payment of $5,000 and the balance of another $5,000 to be paid when the phone lines were installed in my house. Hers was an incoming business, which is why they are known as call girls.

Having taken over Madeleine's empire, the first thing I had to do was reorganize her black book to conform to my own listing system. Her book had hundreds of listings of clients, their price, credit rating, erotic preferences or aberrations, and sometimes even their dimensions. Most of the men, naturally, had aliases or were given them by Madeleine.

Some men were listed by their preference in liquor, such as Red Label, Mr. Cutty, or Mr. Sark. Some invented their own aliases, like Marco Polo, Plato, Aristotle, Caesar, and the more ordinary Mr. White, Mr. Black, Mr. Brown, Mr. Green.

Some of the names these aliases disguised were very famous indeed. The book was such a celebrity-packed register it could make the society columns look like a truck driver's time sheet.

While I had come to be regarded as a friendly and witty madam to the Jewish community, Madeleine was more or less known as a leading lady to the WASPs, so when I took over her business I became a force for religious brotherhood.

Her book was basically made up of "live ones"—which meant men who still actively patronized a brothel, and not some old fuddy-duddies who could no longer get it up. There were exceptions, however, as I found when I called up to advise her clients of the change of management, and I had one or two embarrassing moments.

One man, Mr. Thomson, did not answer his phone, but the creaky, old voice that did said: "This is Mrs. Thomson speaking; Mr. Thomson has been dead for four years."

A Mr. Morris said: "You should have called me up ten years ago. I'm almost seventy-five now, and I can't get it up anymore."

Another man didn't have an age problem, but didn't thank me for calling. "My dear madam," Mr. Purgavie icily informed me, "that number dates back to the days when I was a wild bachelor around town. These days I am a respectable and happily married man, so don't ever call me at home again—but here's my office number."

To those who were receptive to my call, I would speak as follows: "Hi, I'm Xaviera Hollander, I'm from Holland, I'm twenty-five years of age [I'd lie a couple of years], I live in a beautiful three-bedroom apartment in midtown, and I have taken over the management of Madeleine's business because she has retired to have a baby.

"Why don't you drop over for coffee and a chat with us and see if you like the atmosphere? If you do, we would be glad to have you as a guest occasionally."

With Madeleine's names and my enterprise, I made back my original investment in two months.

The book was such a little gold mine that it should have been locked in Fort Knox, but because it was required by the phone at all times to check out a customer's credentials, I could not give it the protection it deserved.

As an indication of how important it is to take care of a book like this, I had a bad experience shortly after I acquired it—because I hired a girl who was managed by a black pimp.

The reason I acted against my better judgment was basically because Roberta was a college graduate, which I found was an interesting attribute for a hooker; she was also clean, pleasant, and attractive in a "Miss Cornfed USA" way.

A week after Roberta started working for me, I had the

opportunity to go out for a leisurely dinner, which is a rare luxury when you become a madam. However, this was a Friday night in the summer, and business was relatively quiet. In charge I left my trustworthy roommate, a working girl named Corinne.

I was gone no more than a couple of hours, but when I returned to the house it was an agitated Corinne who greeted me.

"Come into your room," she whispered. "I have something important to tell you."

She was worried about the honesty of Roberta. "I needed the black book to check out a caller, and discovered it and Roberta were both missing. Your bathroom door was locked for almost an hour, and when Roberta reappeared, so did the book," she told me.

I called Roberta in and accused her point-blank of copying names from my book, which she hastily denied.

"Then how did the book get in the bathroom? Did it grow legs and walk?"

Roberta gave me some unsatisfactory explanation. "I cannot tolerate disloyalty to the house or to the madam," I said, "so I will have to ask you to leave."

The next day her pimp phoned up four times, begging me to take her back. He also sent me two bunches of yellow roses. He realized my house was the best in town, and nowhere else would she make a certain $150 to $200 a night.

Again, against my better judgment, I agreed to give her another chance on the condition that she tighten up her game and not try any further deceit.

A few days later, as I was sitting in my bedroom going over accounts, I could hear the extension phone in the living room being used repeatedly. Normally I would never snoop on my girls, but Roberta was around, and I was no longer sure of her.

Besides, it was my business phone she was tying up. As I lifted the receiver, I heard her talking with another girl.

"Mr. Brennan doesn't seem to know you, Roberta, and he wants more detail," the other girl, also a hooker, was saying. To which Roberta replied, "Just tell him you have been referred by Madam Xaviera."

Not only was it my phone, in my house, but it was also one of my most regular customers. They were obviously both working for the same pimp and trying to approach one of the names she had copied from my black book. I hit the ceiling.

I was so angry I was shaking, and Corinne had to restrain me from going out and throwing her bodily into the street.

"Get dressed, get out, and don't bother to have your pimp send me any yellow roses or make any attempt to contact me ever again!" was my farewell to Roberta.

Thankfully, that kind of dishonesty is unusual, and generally speaking, my girls are very loyal to me. Because of our closeness in ages, we are more like girlfriends than the traditional madam-prostitute relationship.

Whenever I can, I give the girls advice and assistance in both their professional and private lives.

It is known that most madams are bisexual, and I am no exception. Whenever a new girl joins me, I usually take her to bed and teach her some basic tricks of the trade, such as how to suck cock or pussy.

Like most madams, I have my favorites and might tend to give them the pick of the customers or the best work, but each girl is dear to me, and I try always to be fair. I can also say I never cheat my girls like some madams who tell them a customer was a $50 date, when in reality he paid $100 and she kept $75 and gave the girl only $25.

As much as I give them guidance in their professional life, if they require it personally I am there to help, too. Sometimes, if I think it is justified, I offer advice uninvited, as in the case of Sarah, a former employee of Madeleine's and for a while a roommate of mine.

Sarah was a sweet-natured but lazy girl who earned the nickname Dopey because she was forever swallowing uppers and downers. As a result, she was always half-doped and did nothing constructive with her private life. I hated to see such a waste, so I gave her the lecture: "Sarah, I would like to see you take more of an interest in life. Why don't you pick up a book now and again and read it instead of lying around all day?"

As head of the household, occasionally I have to be tough with the girls, and with the customers as well, if one complains about the other.

If a customer tells me that a girl is uncooperative or crude, I call her aside and ask if something is wrong. If more than one man complains, I have to caution her, and if it happens too often, I usually have to let her go.

On the other hand, if a girl complains that a customer is rough or drunk and giving her hard time, I have to handle that, too. All she has to do is slip into one of the bathrooms that adjoin the bedrooms, call me in discreetly, and tell me.

I don't scream insults or get bitchy at men the way Georgette would do with her drunks, or the way Madeleine would do to a man who rejected her. I knock on the bedroom door, respectfully request permission to enter, and tell him the young lady says he is treating her badly.

If I see her complaint is justified, I ask him to dress—or have a massage first if he wants and a coffee—but to leave the premises as soon as possible and come back again next week when he is sober.

The madam herself, generally speaking, is too busy to get involved in any sexual activity unless it is a complicated sado-masochistic scene that perhaps only she is qualified to do. This is especially so now that the complex call-line system has been installed and the client books have all been reorganized to correspond with each of the four different color phones.

So if a man specifically requests to have me and is willing to pay the higher fee, I might go to bed with him, but he has to put up with the phones ringing and me answering them. Sometimes the phone interruptions can be a beautiful tease, and I laugh it off with, "Oh, darling, at least you can't say I've rushed you, because we are going to start all over again."

But if the money was right, and coitus interruptus makes him mad, and he says, "Screw the damn phones," I might consider taking the phones off the hook for a while.

One great privilege of being a madam as opposed to a working girl is that she can choose for herself any customer she would like to go with. If a groovy-looking guy walks in, I can snap him up for myself. The perfect situation I try to engineer is for a great-looking guy to pay for a three-way scene with me and my favorite girl of the moment. That way I get to swing with them both and make more money as well.

Being a successful madam has its liabilities as well as its rewards, as I tell any girl who wants to go into the business. I had to pay a high rent, take care of tips to doormen and chauffeurs, and deal with the salaries of cleaning women and "butlers." The booze bill was colossal, and when a client's check bounced, I still had to pay the girl, while whenever there was a police raid, I was responsible for the legal costs and fines. One of the liabilities is that your time is no longer your own. When a working girl completes her shift, she is free to meet her boyfriend or husband and relax as she likes. When I was working as a single, I took off Wednesday and Saturday nights or went away for a long weekend.

It so happens I love the work I am doing.

Nowadays there are few days off, but if I did not have day-long phone contact with clients and friends, I would probably go crazy.

When fatigue builds up, and I simply have to take a break, I fly off to Miami, Las Vegas, or the Caribbean for a few days—provided I can find a substitute madam to take over for me.

It is almost impossible to find a girl who is smart enough to handle the phones and the customers, sufficiently interested to see that all goes well, but not so ambitious that, in your absence, she will try to take away half the business for herself.

Last July 4, when I intended to go to Curaçao for the long weekend, I had the choice of the Argentine girls who work for me or the Canadian girls, who lived in but who were recent arrivals from Montreal—and I could use none of them. First of all, for some reason, customers don't want to hear a Spanish-accented voice answer the phone. I have no personal prejudices, but to them all Spanish accents are Puerto Rican. As for the Canadian girls, I knew that their dedication to the business did not go beyond making a quick few bucks.

The girl I finally found was Wanda, a professor of art and history at a New York university who had a good head on her shoulders, but whose only ambition in prostitution was to supplement her legitimate earnings by coming over now and again to make a quick hundred, and out.

Wanda was also honest and hardworking, but, as I found out

when I returned, not tough enough. She was not able to control the girls, and I learned that a fight even broke out between a Canadian and an Argentine over which of them should go with one girl.

Also, my books were all upside down and reshuffled. I vowed that the next time I took a trip, I would leave a message on my answering machine that I was away and the house was closed for a couple of days, although that is the surest way of losing business. Customers expect a twenty-four-hour service every day, otherwise they go somewhere else.

Madeleine used to close shop at three in the morning and take the phones off the hook until noon, but many of my men feel my place is their second home and that I am there twenty-four hours a day. Some of them even want to come over for breakfast dates, while many who work in the neighborhood show up for luncheon meetings. Instead of going out to eat, they jump over here and have food sent up. Then I have the cocktail business, which is relatively quiet until 11:00 P.M. The biggest hours are 11:00 to 4:00 A.M., and sometimes later.

One thing I have always missed as a madam is the personal touch I enjoyed when I worked for a madam myself. Whether I was making love by choice or as part of the job, I was able to get close to a man and his problems without the constant distraction of phones and people intruding. As the head of a flourishing call girl operation, I miss the intimacy. My task is to be elegant, a good hostess, to allocate bedrooms and girls, collect money, and to keep things running smoothly.

Once in a while, I have the opportunity to give a "freebie" to a man in his twenties or thirties who does not have to get back to his wife or check in to his hotel. I get him to wait until we shut the shop and sleep over. And how I need that loving! It is a marvelous sensation to be able to talk and listen, and to share a laugh—as well as fucking—without feeling that I have rented my body for half an hour. And anyway, I need my daily orgasm.

But the most satisfying thing is when one of these young men comes back because he wants to sleep with me and is willing to pay for something he had free (and for which I feel like paying *him*!).

No sooner has lover boy departed, than the phones start ringing. Most men wake up with a monstrous erection, sometimes dismissed as a "piss hard-on," and the desire to start the day with a bang. Not the most romantic beginning to my day, but I won't turn down these breakfast dates and if none of the girls is ready, I do the entertaining myself, no matter how active my night before.

Call me mercenary. Or call me madam. As I tell my customers, I don't care, just call me any time!

Ten

The Oldest Profession
Updated, or,
Behind Open Doors

STORY ONE: He's twenty-nine, and he's terrified. He has never been with a woman before, and from the way he trembles, you would think he is going to get circumcised instead of seduced.

The shy, prematurely balding young man in clean, faded jeans was sent to me by a respected New York City psychiatrist. He is one of the many whose sexual hang-ups I have cured.

My method? Basically the same principle as Masters and Johnson, only they charge thousands and it's called therapy. I charge $50 and it's called prostitution.

With this young man, however, I reduced the fee because I have heard he is on a tight budget. He was a recent law-school graduate, attractive, and polite, and I wanted to help him make some girl a nice boyfriend.

To put him at ease, I told him some things about myself, including that I am bisexual. This broke the ice, and he awkwardly confessed something he had not told even his analyst after twelve years in therapy: several years ago he performed fellatio on a college buddy.

To me this was a good sign. The fact he committed the deed indicates he is the aggressor and can more easily be led into a straight life than a passive male.

However, in order to get into his head and find out where his deep tendencies lie, I showed him several books full of erotic pictures of heterosexual and homosexual lovers—male and female—as well as men and women in leather outfits with whips, manacles, and handcuffs. The last he rejects immediately, so that eliminates sadomasochism.

"What turned you on the most, the men's penises or the girls' vaginas?" I asked.

"The men," he said. "I would feel much safer in a homosexual relationship because it doesn't represent such a big responsibility and obligation." But he did not particularly care for the gay bars, the transvestites, or the superficiality of cruising guys for mere physical relief.

"Tell me," I asked, "did you find the women repulsive?"

"Not at all," he said.

"Then let's go into the bedroom, shall we?" The young man followed me like he was going to the gallows, and once inside, sat down in a chair with his hands unconsciously going to his lap to protect his threatened virtue. His knees still shook a little.

"Why don't you take off your tie and jacket and relax while I slip into the bathroom," I suggested, and left the room to freshen and perfume myself with some sweet lotions. But when I returned five minutes later, clad in a scant orange towel, he was still glued to the chair.

The seduction would have to be mine. Softly I started kissing his neck and blowing suggestive words into his ears as I removed his jacket, shirt, and tie.

"I don't know what you're doing to me," he sort of stammered, "but I never felt this kind of feeling before." Goose bumps came out on his chest and arms.

I happen to get turned on by seducing young virgin boys, and my heart was really in my work. I slowly revealed my body by letting the towel drop to the floor; I lay down on the bed under the circular ceiling mirror and started stroking my body. "It looks like a wonderful movie in the mirror," I whispered. "Come over and look with me."

Bashfully he removed the rest of his clothes and lay down too. The undulating images in the golden glass so turned him on that he reached for his glasses to get a better view.

"Please let me do that to you," he said, and clumsily began stroking my breasts. Then he started sucking them, which was kind of funny—not at all well done, but certainly well meant. So I taught him how to caress a woman's breasts and where to go with his tongue to give her the most pleasure. I did the same to him, and his nipples stood up erect. Dread had been replaced by desire.

Gently I rolled the young man over, straddling his back with my knees on either side and my breasts pressed against him, and nibbled his back gently from his neck down to his buttocks.

There are certain erogenous zones on a man's or woman's back, which, if given little chews, send an electric vibration straight to the sexual organ. When I turned my patient back over, he had a beautiful erection. I gave the same kisses to the front of his body, working down from his temples, neck, chest, and around the pubic triangle to his balls. I started kissing them, putting each in my mouth, but not for too long, because some men, especially when they are under thirty, are ticklish and will laugh and lose their erection.

Then I took his penis like it was a delicious ice-cream cone and slid my tongue over the ice cream. Wow! That wigged him out! But I didn't suck him for long, because I could sense the tension building in his cock, and I knew if I kept it up he would ejaculate, with the most important part of the treatment yet to come.

The first position I chose for lovemaking was spoon fashion— me on my side and him curling around me, and I slipped him into me that way. Then, without letting his penis leave my body, I got on my knees, and we continued doggy style. That way he slipped out a few times, because it is a complicated position for a beginner.

He was enjoying it tremendously, and after thirty minutes was still keeping it up, and I was glad the phone hadn't rung, which it usually does every ten minutes. However, I could tell the finale was near.

In order to let him penetrate deeper for the paradise stroke, I lay over on my back with a silk pillow under my hips and my ankles over his shoulders, and that way, panting and bathed in perspiration, he climaxed.

"I never knew making love to a woman could be so beautiful," he said when he was dressed and ready to leave.

"I think you are cured, and I'm glad. However, I was the aggressor today, but from now on it is up to you. Don't be afraid of women, just try to find the type you like, and act like a man, not like a baby. And good luck."

STORY TWO: I strike up a conversation with a couple on the beach in Puerto Rico, and a Mrs. Katz starts telling me how nice it is, you know, to have a vacation with her husband while her mother-in-law stays home in New Jersey and takes care of the kids.

She is obviously the type who never goes out because she enjoys staying in Cabbageville, raising the family—Mrs. Average Housewife.

But her husband, who is a garment-district executive, sure looks like a bon vivant. I know he is a typical john because while she was away buying an ice cream, he put my card in the pocket of his beach jacket and said, "I can't do anything here, but I'll call you when I get back to New York." While he is chatting with his buddies, I strike up a conversation with her.

So I touch on the subject of love and marriage with Mrs. Katz.

"Mrs. Katz, if your husband needed a harmless little bit of variety once in a while, and if you had the choice, would you prefer he was unfaithful with a hooker and paid her fifty dollars or hundred dollars and came home happy just an hour late once or twice a month? Or would you prefer he found a mistress, set her up in an apartment, perhaps bought her a mink coat? And instead of taking you to Jamaica or Puerto Rico, he took her?"

Now, I don't look like a hooker, I think. I am as brown as a peanut, my hair is streaked blond by the sun and combed neatly to my shoulders, and I look more like a Nordic-type tourist.

"He's better off with a prostitute," Mrs. Katz sighed. So I smile, and she looks at me, and I think she guesses.

STORY THREE: Robert is a handsome, rich, and very successful twenty-eight-year-old investment banker who recently married a girl he had been dating for six months. He loved her very much and really treated her like a queen.

But after only three weeks of marriage, her whole family started moving in on his money. Why don't you buy her these stocks? Why don't you set up this fund? Why don't you put the new house in her name?

And although he really adored her, he realized she loved only his money, and he walked out.

Robert could not afford to be seen dating other girls around town, or his wife's grasping family would really sock it to him financially, so he came to my house.

"I'm not the kind of guy to be hustled for my money," he said the first night. However, he did not quibble about the staggering tab for the several girls he had, and I am sure had I demanded it, he would have paid more. But I am not the type to put my hands around a man's wallet and squeeze. Besides, he was so groovy that even if he were broke I would have let him go for free. He was happy to pay for his pleasure. "I would much rather spend my money on a bunch of prostitutes who are more honest than my wife and at least give me my money's worth," he said.

So a contemporary brothel must be many things to many people, and for many reasons.

It is obvious what it is to most! A pay-for-play parlor, but believe it or not, some even use my house not to get laid!

Still others come because a discreet prostitute is the only person to whom they dare expose the sexual hang-ups they conceal from their wives and girlfriends to avoid creating a scandal.

A statistic that surprises most people is the percentage of eligible bachelors who patronize my house, when, in this day of sexual liberation, there is so much free stuff around.

The fact that the single man turns up mostly after 11:00 P.M. is testimony in itself as to why he came.

He has taken a girl on a date, wined and dined her, enjoyed her company, been turned on, made the eternal overture, and she has responded with some unflattering excuse such as "I have to go home and wash my hair" or "I have to get up very early."

His ardor for her dimmed, but his appetite not sated, he takes out his black book and calls his favorite madam or call girl, and for less money than the cost of his evening out, in most cases, he can discharge his desires without any hassle.

Married men, who make up the largest slice of brothel business, come for a variety of reasons. Geographically they may be out-of-town businessmen, or perhaps recently separated or divorced and not yet fixed up with a new girlfriend. Others are wanting the exotic and unusual that they don't see at home and are fed up with D.I.B. (dead-in-bed) wives who just lie there like starfish.

Whatever it is a man is looking for, a good madam should be able to come up with the goods.

What happens when a man walks through a brothel door? Let me take you on a guided tour of my house, explain a few trade secrets, explode a few old myths, and try to establish the fact that a modern brothel no longer deserves the title house of ill fame or ill repute, but house of pleasure.

On any weekday night there are five to ten girls on hand to entertain the customers, to say nothing of my book listing three hundred better-class hookers in the city who can be called in. That is not to say the house is like a sex supermarket; it is more like a boutique where exclusivity and good taste prevail.

Mine is an international establishment, full of birds of different plume. I have blondes, brunettes, redheads, Scandinavians, Eurasians, American Indians, Negroes, and several South American girls from Chile, Ecuador, and Argentina. The latter are famous for their big boobs and their love of sex. The Scandinavian girls, outwardly cool, are often bright and passionate.

With girls like this, a man from any corner of the world can walk through my door and be welcomed in his own language. I personally speak English, French, German, Spanish, Italian, Dutch, Afrikaans, and some Yiddish.

On entering our calling, the girls usually choose a professional name for themselves, dropping their last name and adopting names like Red Peril, Rainbow, Blondie, Mia Cara, Teardrop, April, May, June; and one girl was even called Shan-da-Lear (as in "swinging from").

The girls who work for me are expected to obey house rules when it comes to dress. Outmoded is the old idea that a brothel is a collection of girls all semidressed in baby-doll pajamas or their underwear. This to me represents a sleazy atmosphere, and the only one permitted to wear a negligee is myself. This is always an expensive figure-fitting Pucci or something similar from the best stores like Saks Fifth Avenue or Bergdorf Goodman.

However, my rules aren't nearly as strict as those of the most famous house in the world, Madam Claude's in Paris, where the girls are expected to look immaculate all the time. Madam Claude, whose girls are dispatched as far east as Beirut and as far west as London, insists her girls buy their clothes from certain couturiers and are coiffed at certain hairdressers. She, no doubt, gets her own kickbacks from these places.*

My girls aren't given strict guidelines on what to wear, but rather what not to wear. I don't want flashy, whorish clothes in

---

*Madame Claude retired to the U.S.A. after running afoul of the French tax authorities in 1974.

the house. Look like a whore and you'll be treated like one is my belief.

I try to set an example in appearance for the girls, and I come on as natural as possible. I wear little makeup, and my hair is always hanging loosely to my shoulders, and always shiny clean. I try to make the natural atmosphere clear through my personality, and not so much through my looks, although my looks are good enough, I suppose. I don't cover them up with artificial eyelashes, wigs, and false nails as a lot of girls do. I seldom wear nail varnish, except on my toes.

I look like a fresh, contemporary girl, which is one of the reasons I do pretty well. My personality is what counts, and this is one of the things that distinguishes one house from another: the personality of the madam. And that is also why I am careful never to hire a girl with a stronger personality.

As far as the girls' choice of dress goes, they usually decide on something to flatter their particular physical attributes: a décolleté gown for a girl whose best feature is her bosom, hot pants or miniskirts for a girl who has great legs, and so on.

Hot pants are big with men, because legs turn them on. Surprisingly enough, when a man comes into a brothel, he doesn't seem to care much what the girl's face looks like. Obviously, he's not going to make a grab at one who looks like the Bride of Frankenstein, but to a customer, boobs, bottoms, and legs—in that order—are more important.

Age, of course, is another factor in a man's choice of bed companion. Somewhere along the line, most men think prostitutes should all be nineteen or twenty years old. A girl can deceive them a few years, but you can't claim a woman who is thirty-one is twenty-one. It doesn't work.

Men in their late twenties to forties don't mind a slightly older girl, so long as she has a nice personality.

I have one girl working for me, Carol, who is thirty-six and the mother of two teenagers. Carol is well read, cheerful, and intelligent—and genuinely loves men, and they can see it. American men crave affection from prostitutes, and Carol knows how to give it to them. If a bashful man walks in, she puts him at ease by taking him to the bar, charms him, then guides him into bed. They seem to forget this girl is not eighteen, but twice that age. Of course, the soft lighting in the living room helps, too. She combines motherly feelings with great femininity.

A lot of customers have a problem choosing a girl, either out of shyness or because they are overwhelmed at the possibilities for selection. If that happens, it is up to me. I stand near him at the bar in a slinky outfit and chat him up for a while as he gets a drink, then I gently put my hands on his leg at the inner thigh to put him at ease, and turn him on a little, then ask, "Would you like to make your choice?"

Some are too bashful or don't wish to embarrass the girl, so they will call me on the side and say, "May I have the redhead sitting on the couch?" Or, "I like the girl in the white blouse."

Sometimes a hayseed from Chattanooga, Tennessee, is too confused to make a suggestion, so I make it for him. For me, making the decision is sometimes difficult, because all the girls are equally nice and dear to me, and I hate to favor one over the other.

However, the girls who live in and pay rent have priority over the callers.

On the other hand, a hooker can reject a man if he is impossibly drunk or looks like Quasimodo. Professional women do not usually get turned off by looks. What most often causes trouble is the man's behavior—or misbehavior.

When a choice is made, one way or the other, I bring the man to the girl and tell her "Give him a guided tour of the house" or "Take him to the mirror room or the bedroom." We never say things like "Give it to him," or, as my first madam, Pearl, said, "Here he is, baby, fuck him."

I always try to give a touch of class to my establishment.

Another rule of the house is the level of conversation in front of customers. I don't want customers alluded to as "tricks," "johns," or "suckers."

Forbidden, too, is talk about money. Sometimes girls get carried away at the big money they are making and start comparing notes in front of the customers.

I have some girls who have come in as shy little secretaries making $130 per week on the outside and think it's great at first to earn $50 to $100 extra a night. As they become more successful in the field, they unfortunately become more competitive and greedy.

This occasionally leads to talk of "How much did you make?"

One cute little button I hired named Lynn, who came from Queens, became so money hungry that she was rushing men in and out of the bedroom and clicking away like a cash register. "I'll suck your cock in the bathroom," I heard her say when the bedrooms were full, and indeed, she got away with it. But in general, a man prefers more for his money.

I like my girls to act ladylike and not like whores.

However, I distinguish between the words *prostitute* and *whore*. My girls are the former.

A prostitute is a girl who knows how to make a man feel good even if he is underendowed, a lousy lover, four feet tall, and has a face only a mother could love. In that case, she should fake it and let him enjoy what he pays for. A good lady of the night is an actress!

Speaking for myself, I try to always give warmth and tenderness and make a man feel like a king or a baby, whichever he wants, even though he is a cash customer.

A whore, on the other hand, takes but doesn't give—unless it is a small souvenir like V.D. or herpes.

How does a girl behave in the bedroom? That is a matter of decision between her and her customer, within reason and within his budget.

I make the girls understand that this is not some kind of Arthur Murray's Dance Studio, where it is a cut-and-dried case of who leads and who follows. If she has never sucked a cock before, I show her some of my home movies, which also give a good course in eating pussy, in case a customer wants to watch that kind of a scene before going himself. Or I take her with me in a threesome and show her how to do it. Most men have fantasies of making love to two girls at once.

A man mostly wants to relax here and be attended rather than attend. For that reason, he will often lie back and ask the girl to do the work, which actually suits professional ladies because it makes less of a demand of their bodies.

However, a girl can't aggressively promote this position, or a man might say "Let me call the shots—I'm paying the freight."

Highest on the list of preferences, after straight sex, is what is called in the trade a blow job, or fellatio.

If a girl comes to me unskilled in this technique, I teach her how to do it on a banana. How to go with her vibrating tongue just under the head, where the skin is sensitive. And I must say, speaking for myself, I simply love to suck cock. I don't enjoy it if he is a boring blow job, as we call them, one who just lies back and doesn't writhe or moan.

Another request is for Greek style—that is, anal sex. If the man makes his desires in this direction known to the madam beforehand, he can be put to bed with a specialist. My Greek-style girl is a slim, pale American blonde who digs it no other way, despite warnings from her gynecologist to lay off, as it were, or risk having her sphincter muscles loosen up.

Around-the-world, or analingus, is another popular request, but, needless to say, not every girl wants to accommodate this desire unless she can diplomatically coax a man into the bath first and scrub up his rectum good. With this technique, men usually don't insist if the girl says it turns her off to suck his ass, balls, and cock.

On the other hand, some men expect to be taken not only around the world but also to the far side of the moon and back for their money.

There are those who want ten different positions, and their general expression is "I want my money's worth," because to them $50 represents a stiff fee, so to speak. A funny thing about these types is that many of them want to eat pussy but practically never kiss a girl on the lips, even when they are coming.

What a girl does depends on the amount of time she has, or sometimes the appeal the man has for her.

Some customers are so nice you want to give them the world on a silver platter. I recently had such a man.

This man, Kenneth, was so delicious, with a beautiful body, but had been screwed up by bad sex. He was about thirty-two years old, married to a very square woman, and he had never fooled around or seen a prostitute until he came to us. The man's looks and manners turned me on.

Even though he was clean, I had in mind something special to do with him, so I suggested we take a shower together, and I washed him up, back, forward, upside down, until he was squeaky clean.

Then I took him to bed and started to make real love to him, starting at the toes, sucking each one as though it were a cock.

Then I began kissing and sucking from his toes up to his legs and his knees, at the same time that I was crawling all over his body with my fingers.

I worked my way up to his balls, which I sucked one at a time; while my fingers went to the bridge between his balls and his rectum, a caress that he loved.

Then I lifted his ass and went in with my tongue. He had never had this done to him, and he flipped out of his mind. He was so beautiful, responsive, and clean. I was going deeper and deeper with my tongue, and his cock and his balls too were going up and down, he was so excited.

Then I put a little jelly on my index finger and put it in his ass, just a little bit, and I could feel that he got very tense. The ass is much like a vagina—a warm opening to put a finger or a cock in.

Then I took my hand away from his rectum, turned him gently over, and gave him a back rub. I teased him with my tongue from the top of his neck to his bottom.

Now on his back once more, I tied a little tourniquet of surgical tubing around the head of his cock. This technique delays a man's orgasm. You tie a piece of surgical tubing, or venetian-blind cord, around the head of his organ, but after he has a hard-on, because otherwise the blood can't get through. The tourniquet stops the blood from circulating, so the balls get really big, and the cock stays up, and he cannot climax.

While I had him this way, I greased up a little vibrator and put it in his ass at the same time as I started sucking his cock, and with all that going on, he nearly went bananas!

After I had almost driven this gorgeous man crazy, I pulled off the tourniquet and made love to him, first doggy style; then with my legs around his shoulders; and finally tree style, with him standing beside the bed while I hung on to his broad shoulder like climbing a tree. I gently put his big cock into my vagina, and a bit awkwardly we climaxed.

On the matter of orchestrating a climax, there is a professional secret to delay premature ejaculation, too. If a girl is sympathetic to the man's problem, she can give him a tube of Detane and tell him to rub some into the head of his penis. It will be sure to slow him down. Sometimes I use a psychological approach, like jokingly telling him to think of his mother-in-law if I sense he is going to explode too soon.

Usually, though, the reverse is the problem: to make a man climax when the meter is running over.

I had one situation where everybody was screwing, but nobody seemed to reach their climax, and my German girl, the resourceful Grethe, worked out a solution.

I sent Grethe as captain of a couple of girls to participate in a bachelor party a group of rich, young men-about-town were holding in the penthouse at the New York Hilton.

When my girls arrived, they found a wild scene in progress, with a band and dancing on the ground floor, and several bedrooms filled with young couples copulating in various positions.

Grethe and my girls sat by, quietly talking to their partners and awaiting their turn on the beds. However, after half an hour nothing was happening except a lot of quiet swishing around going on.

Grethe grew restless and decided to hurry them up by staging a sexy atmosphere. On the same principle that one makes noise like running water to encourage urination, Grethe started puffing, panting, groaning, and simulating orgasm sounds, and within five minutes everybody was doing the same. Then the first session of girls all ran to the bathroom to wash up, and my girls and their partners hopped into bed.

Needless to say, hygiene is a very important aspect of the profession on everyone's part. A girl doesn't want to do all kinds of intimate things with a man who is not fresh, and the reverse is true, too. Since I sell girls, I make sure they know all about shaving their underarms and legs, using lotions, bathing, and douching. A professional girl should be able to douche at least twice a day without exceeding a danger limit and risk drying the sensitive internal tissue.

To protect herself against infection, a girl tries to look at a man's penis before he goes to the bathroom and has the chance to urinate, thereby concealing traces of disease. However, in a house like mine, this danger does not occur.

If a man wants protection for himself, he will ask for a rubber, which I willingly supply.

Once or twice I have had a customer who behaved like a kid in a candy store, having several girls in a session, and the unaccustomed activity caused a strain resulting in a slight discharge.

However, in my two years as a professional, whether it is luck, my selectivity in both men and women, or the result of hygiene vigilance, I have never come across a case of venereal disease. I maintain that it is the little freebies giving it away in the First Avenue bars or on student campuses who spread this hazard.

I am known to be obsessively clean, and the first thing I notice about a person is his or her fingernails. I drag a man over to the sink and scrub his hands if he looks grubby.

Careful as I am, early in my career I caught a little devil

called crabs. At the first itch, I took myself off to the gynecologist to be checked out.

She was a dear old motherly type who probed around, located the demon, and took it on a slide to the microscope, where she confirmed my suspicions.

"My goodness," she said, "a crabbie, dear." Then she added apologetically, "I don't want to alarm you, but have you been with a man you don't know very well lately?"

Obviously I changed gynecologists and found somebody a little more broad-minded and equipped to understand the problems of a working girl.

The man I found is the "trade" specialist, a groovy man with a practice near fashionable Fifth Avenue in the Seventies. This man is to prostitutes what a trainer is to professional football players. He keeps in good playing condition all the muscles and tissues and tubes that in our trade get overworked and sometimes abused.

Although it is a myth that professional girls rush to their gynecologist for semiweekly checkups, whenever we have a problem, Dr. Jonathan Sayer, as I'll call him, is the man we go to.

He is a good doctor, broad-minded, who devotes a lot of time to each patient, and his prices are fair: $50 for the first visit and $25 thereafter.

He is also the first doctor I have come across in this country with whom it is possible to be alone. Unlike in Europe, doctors here have you all bundled up in gowns and tied with strings and presented like a gift-wrapped package, with the nurse looking on like a hawk.

Dr. Sayer, however, sees you alone, and while his bedside manner is devastating, as far as I know he has never made a pass at a patient, despite many of their attempts to persuade him to do so.

Several girls, I understand, who have fallen on lean times have asked to pay their bills in trade, but he has politely declined. One lovestruck patient, recognizing that she would never get him into bed, bought him a bullwhip one Christmas and pleaded, "Doctor, just beat me up a little, please."

How do professionals protect themselves against pregnancy and other occupational hazards? How do they overcome the unproductive four-day period?

Most girls prefer to protect themselves by using the Pill, although some use a diaphragm. This useful little gadget is also a professional trick for holding back the menstrual flow.

The way we do it is to douche thoroughly first, insert the diaphragm, then douche again to remove traces of blood and the vaginal jelly, and it is impossible to detect that a girl is in that time of the month.

Although this effectively holds back the flow, this method gives you only half an hour's respite and has to be removed immediately.

Some girls overcome the four-day inconvenience by using large wads of cotton. I do not recommend this method because a strong partner can push the cotton to regions from which only a gynecologist can retrieve it.

A so-called hygienic sponge on a string is another handy gadget that serves the same purpose and, unlike the cotton, retains its cohesion. The string is hidden in the girl's rectum.

One of the working girl's best friends is a product called Koromex jelly, or KY. This violet-flavored lubricant will ease the way when passion does not. That is to say, if a girl has spent her natural lubrication or is not turned on by a man, a little lubricant helps out. Too much friction can injure a girl's vagina.

Who are prostitutes, and how did they get into the business in the first place?

A lot of them are part-time models or actresses failed in their ambitions or waiting to realize them.

Many are dyed-in-the-wool whores who have known no other gainful employment. On the other hand, many girls come into the business for a specific amount of time to make quick money and then split.

Only stupid girls are likely to hang on in this business until they are forty or worn-out or pregnant or drug users and don't know what to do anymore.

I admire the girl who is smart enough and has sufficient willpower and resistance to get out after she has made a killing, and keep a straight job with less money.

Two examples are Gayle and Gilda, both very intelligent girls and both knowing exactly what they wanted from the business.

Gayle got out when she married a very nice account executive from a big ad agency. She thanked me for helping her earn the money that made it possible to attract her man, and moved out to Westchester County with her husband.

However, three months later she was on the phone again saying her husband was gambling two nights a week, and she needed extra money to pay some of his debts; also, she didn't dig sitting around at home doing nothing. She came out and worked for a while, but vanished when her husband gave up his gambling.

Gilda was working for a big brokerage house on Wall Street when her boyfriend got involved with the Mafia bad guys and was in debt to the tune of several grand.

Gilda, who had absolutely no head for prostitution and was basically very square, indeed prudish, turned out to be a great

$200 dinner date whom men took on social-business dinners. She came to me knowing exactly what she wanted, and after earning it, left again. She had what I called willpower, because when I have called her up since to offer her a quick $50 or $100, she has refused.

Some little rich kids get into the business for kicks or out of a desire to be rebellious, and in my experience they get out quick and marry the guy back home whom they ran away from in the first place.

There is a saying that prostitutes make the best wives. This to me is definitely a myth.

Such a woman never seems to be capable of sharing the rest of her life with just one man, no matter how well he takes care of her. Madeleine herself, while still young, had gone through three husbands, and each time she split, she would drift back into prostitution. And once she was running a prosperous bordello, she would not easily be tempted away. Only pregnancy or tax problems would send her scurrying back into matrimony. Prostitutes often start as nymphomaniacs, but after staying too long in the business end up hating men. They can't settle down and always want more action—or more money. So whenever I am asked the inevitable question, What's a nice girl like you doing in a job like this? I think seriously about getting married, and I have turned down some pretty good offers.

But there is something about the call-girl world which appeals to me: the variety of interesting men one meets, the independence of running my own business, and it was not as if I were genuinely in love. So, when trade was booming, why give it up for life in the suburbs, security, and so-called respectability? Not me, not for all the fur coats, not even for a baby.

Eleven

Different Strokes for Different Folks, or, Wall Street and Me

9've got a friend at Chase Manhattan, Barclays, First National City, Franklin National, Marine Midland, the Dime, Greenwich Bank and Trust, the Bowery, Manufacturers Hanover, Bankers Trust, the New York Bank for Savings, the Bank of America, the Bank of Israel, the Bank of Tokyo, and just about every other bank, major or minor, operating in this country.

In other words, bankers are among my very best customers.

These money men account for about 10 percent of my business, and when you consider the dozens of other professional categories—from athletes to aristocrats, doctors to diplomats, publishers to politicians, lawyers to judges, company presidents and other businessmen and even some movie stars and clergy—all patronizing my house, this occupation makes up a substantial share of the market.

There is only one other profession that outranks bankers as dedicated clients, and that is the stockbroker. These are such a horny bunch of brothel-creepers that I would estimate 50 percent of my business is directly tied to the market trends.

If the averages take a significant tumble, the stockbrokers will not!

Happily, the reverse is true, and if it has been a good day on Wall Street, I can be certain that by eleven o'clock that night my phone will ring red hot, or groups of six or eight juiced-up stockbrokers will appear at my door. When the stocks go up, the cocks go up!

Brokers, as a group, are likelier to patronize my premises, whereas the more conservative bankers tend frequently to call up for take-out service. But no matter where, when, how, or why their desire, I always go out of my way to satisfy their demands, because if I don't, there is generally a rival madam who will.

One relatively quiet Friday night this summer I received a late-late call from a regular New York banker customer wanting six girls for the same number of out-of-town investment bankers he was entertaining. It happened that the girls who were not otherwise professionally occupied were already away for the weekend or enjoying their boyfriends' company, so in order not to let the bankers down, I decided to take on the assignment by myself.

I was pleased to discover when I went over to the Hilton that they were all staying on the same floor and had appointed their New York host as treasurer, so it was just a matter of negotiating with him a package deal and zipping from one room to the next—boom, boom, fifteen minutes, in, out—and I was back home in two hours considerably richer.

Another time I took it upon myself to attend a mortgage bankers convention in Miami to further my goodwill, and, naturally, increase my wealth.

On that occasion last winter, I took along one of my stronger girls, Raquel, and checked into the Fontainebleau, where the convention was being held. During the day we would sit by the pool soaking up the warm sun and engaging in social chitchat, while, all the time, I kept my eyes open to see which cabanas the bankers occupied.

On the first afternoon, we squeezed in a couple of customers before our late-afternoon nap, and after dinner that night we made our pitch in the Poodle Lounge, where the delegates were all together. I would start up a conversation about being down from New York, and the banker would usually ask, "And what are you doing here in Miami?"

"I am here for entertainment purposes," I would answer.

"Are you a singer or a dancer or something like that?"

"No," I would reply, "I am here to entertain the mortgage bankers." It was as simple and direct as that, and to show you what good customers they were, the first night we had about six men each, and the second night, after word spread like a brushfire, I remember going up and down in the hotel elevator ten times in less than three hours.

Business was so fantastic that we didn't have the strength to last the four-day convention. On the fourth morning, I woke up so exhausted that I told Raquel, "Pack your bags, we're flying back to New York today."

At home in my own house I could earn the same money as administrator while my girls did the strenuous work. However, I believe I built up several lasting contacts in Miami, because many of these bankers still call me whenever they are in New York.

I first gained my good reputation with the stockbrokers in my fledgling days when I operated alone in my little studio and was known to be able to take on half a dozen at one time. While I would be screwing one, the others would be lining up in the kitchen, boozing and joking. The more I screwed, the hornier I became, so that everybody went away happy, and we all had a lot of laughs as well.

With bankers, and especially brokers, it is important that they are given a scrupulously honest financial deal, because if one of them felt cheated out of his money's worth, word could spread along Wall Street, and you could lose a slice of your business.

Brokers, while they may be my biggest customers, are not necessarily my favorite ones, especially when they arrive at my house polluted and rowdy and arguing about who goes with whom and for how much. The loud behavior of this particular raucous type, I believe, is a reflection of their ethnic origins, because most of them are of Irish descent.

Last St. Patrick's Day my house was like Belfast under siege. They arrived in drunken groups, and I had a difficult time keeping order, with them running around wearing nothing but green neckties or bright green ribbons around their cocks, boozing and carrying on more than they were using my girls.

I will say one thing for the Irish-American stockbroker types, though—they are always horny, and even if the market dips, they still want to come around. But they try to get away for less money.

In a bordello, certain ethnic groups tend to conform to a pattern, and I have compiled what I term Madam Xaviera's Dirty Dozen.

ITALIAN-AMERICANS run a close second to the IRISH for sexual exuberance, but unlike the latter, they rarely quarrel about the price, and they are more choosy about their girls, usually preferring blondes.

AMERICAN JEWS are my favorite and most frequent customers. They have a wonderful sense of humor, behave themselves, and treat the girls with consideration. Often they really appreciate a good blow job, and I wonder if that is not because their fastidious wives would not stoop to smear their lipsticks. So prostitutes usually agree that they are appreciative and undemanding.

But not always. I remember a Mr. Appelbaum who complained to me that his wife was as cold as a dead fish. It was his first time in my house, and he was both nervous and excited. I started to undress, but before I could finish, he had jumped on top of me, rammed his stiff little prick inside me, and after three or four thrusts collapsed like a sack of potatoes.

"That was great!" he enthused. "Did you come too?"

"Mr. Appelbaum, that was not lovemaking but *schtupping* [a Yiddish term for hard fucking]. No wonder you think your wife is frigid; how do you think that she could ever get warmed up by somebody who is faster than a rabbit?"

He was astonished. He had taken his sex problem to a psychiatrist, but after a few more sessions with me, he was able to give up the shrink, and his marriage blossomed. A good hooker can be a first-class social worker, but I don't suppose that Mrs. Appelbaum ever realized that I was her husband's therapist.

Sometimes the celebrated Jewish guilt took curious forms. I was visited by an extremely handsome young man, his wedding ring prominently displayed. When I went to kiss him, he turned his face away. Bad breath? I took his cock in my mouth, and as we both grew excited, I turned myself so that my crotch, warm and wet, was well within range of his tongue. But, again no dice!

Finally, I begged him to fuck me; I was missing out on my daily orgasm, but he shook his head.

"You see," he explained, "with my cock inside your mouth, I don't feel guilty, but if I were to kiss or fuck you, that really would be cheating."

GREEKS. On a private basis, young Greek men are the ones I adore most as lovers. They are sensitive, strong, warm, and exciting. Greeks are rarely circumcised, but they are very clean. The older, richer Greeks as customers are very charming and sophisticated in bed, and sometimes slightly kinky. They tend to prefer anal sex, a taste which I believe they acquired in the days when their girls were expected to be virgins when they married, and yet their hot Greek blood dictated otherwise. To overcome this technicality, they invented what is known professionally as Greek style, and the men still enjoy it that way today.

Then there are the BRITISH. They tend to be civilized, skillful, and a trifle cold. I suppose their taste for masochism results from their so-called public school education, and they bring their class consciousness into the brothel with them. Once they have finished, and their account is settled, they shake hands and depart, and never stop to mingle with lesser mortals. As for the DUTCH, I have to confess that my fellow countrymen are the world's most unromantic and unimaginative lovers. They flop on top of you, nearly squeezing the air out of your lungs, do their dull Dutch thing, and then sit about for hours, chattering among themselves and drinking your booze.

I have mixed feelings about the FRENCH. They certainly know what to do with their tongues, and it is no coincidence that the whole world uses the French term for *soixante-neuf*: 69. But their ideas on personal hygiene often do not measure up to my standards, although I find them cute lovers if I can coax them into the tub before the bed. The GERMANS are clean enough, but robust rather than romantic and at times downright dictatorial. "You will now open the legs!" comes the peremptory command, and I find it wise to keep those types well away from my Jewish clients, especially the ISRAELIS. Unlike the American Jews, these Israeli-born *sabras* are assertive and macho. They are virile and like to give head to women, without any trace of the proverbial guilt.

For sheer charm, give me the HUNGARIANS and the AUSTRI-ANS. Well mannered and sophisticated, these gentlemen from the Europe of old-world operettas never fail to bring a little present when they come to my establishment. My ITALIAN and SPANISH customers are great lovers, elegant dressers, and they prefer to take a pretty and intelligent girl to the most expensive restaurants and nightclubs instead of merely getting laid.

LATIN AMERICANS (including Mexicans). In general, they are lovers rather than customers. They don't mind spending their money, but they believe their $100 buys them the girl for the whole night. To them it's not the money that matters, but they don't want to be rushed. If I send a girl to a hotel to see, for example, a Texan, I know she will be back in three quarters of an hour, because as far as pay-for-play goes, American men know the score. However, if I send her over to see a Latin American, she'll be gone at least two hours.

The Latins want to romance the girl in their slow Occidental English, which is very time-consuming. They are like big children in their way, but very nice, charming, and appreciative just the same.

To give you an example of their behavior in a brothel, I will tell the story of what happened earlier this year when I closed my house one Friday night at the request of a South American minister of finance and three of his country's most prominent bankers. I assured the minister that except for his party and their two girls apiece, nobody else would be allowed on the premises. However, sitting around idly while they were all going in and out of the bedrooms made me very horny, so when a very sexy friend of mine, Takis, a Greek boy, called up, I invited him over.

When Takis arrived, the bedrooms were all occupied, so we had no alternative but to make love on the living-room sofa, and to hell with my promise not to let anyone else in. Although the Latins did say "no other customers," this doesn't necessarily mean "no lovers."

After we made passionate love for about half an hour, I became aware that the minister of finance and his party had trickled out of the bedrooms and taken ringside seats with their girlfriends to watch the madam putting on an impromptu exhibition.

It occurred to me they had a right to be mad at my entertaining another man, but that was not so. When we finally needed a rest, the Latins gave us a standing ovation, grinning broadly and shouting, "Bravo! Bravo!"

Charming, and sometimes childlike as they are, Latin men stubbornly refuse to go with Latin women, at least in a brothel.

ORIENTALS. We have a saying that going to bed with an Oriental is like washing your hands: clean and simple. These men are the quickest lovers and the smallest in dimensions. They are so quick and easy to take care of that when the new Chinese restaurant opened recently in my building, I arranged to have regular meals sent up to my house in exchange for a monthly screw for every man on the staff, even the cook. Noodles for doodles, you might call it.

As far as Oriental clients go, Japanese patronize brothels much more than Chinese, the latter being a more discreet, private race of people.

Many Oriental men are painfully aware of their physical shortcomings and will go to bizarre lengths to conceal or compensate for them.

I once had a poignant experience in a hotel room with a high-class Japanese man who could not face up to the reality of the size of his equipment.

The man, a minister of the Japanese cabinet, visiting New York, was lying in the darkened room with the covers pulled over him when I arrived at the request of his American male secretary.

As my eyes became accustomed to the dark, I could see that he was in his early forties and quite attractive. He didn't say much, so I undressed quickly and joined him in his bed, assuming he would leave all the action up to me.

However, in bed, when I tried to go down on him, he gently but firmly pushed my head away. At first I thought this might be coyness on his part, but he kept pushing me away until he saw I was so determined to suck his cock that he allowed me to.

But he refused to remove his hands from where they were covering his balls and holding on to the base of his penis. At first I thought he was doing this to hold it up for me, but after awhile I began to realize that there was something very strange about the penis I was sucking. The skin was not as soft as on a real cock, and when I went to put the point of my tongue into the little eye, I couldn't find one.

Something, I knew, was very weird in that bed. But before I could find out, he rolled me onto my back, made quick love, climaxed in minutes, and vanished into the bathroom.

If I had not felt myself warm and wet when I reached down under the sheets, I would have suspected the man was wearing an artificial penis. It didn't make sense.

Five minutes later when he returned from the bathroom, with his hands still covering his front, I had made no attempt to get up and get dressed. I wanted to get to the bottom of this, so to speak.

The Japanese cabinet minister slid back under the sheets and started talking with me in polite, labored English, and as he did I gently pushed his hand away and found, to my amazement, a penis not even as big as my little finger.

I believe if he had been a Caucasian and the lights had been on, I would have seen that man blush crimson at that moment.

"How come you were shaped so well five minutes ago?" I asked him. "Did you wear something over your penis?"

"Never mind, never mind," he said. "Everything okay now."

"Tell me the truth," I coaxed. "I will understand, honestly."

There was no point in pretending, so he admitted to me he had indeed worn an artificial penis, which, I have since found out, is quite commonplace in Japan. It is such an ingenious little device that it can be controlled to simulate orgasm at the same time as the wearer and squirt out a semenlike liquid.

"Listen," I said to him. "There is no need to be ashamed of your real penis. And to prove it, I will suck it again for you." This time he let me do it, and I believe he really enjoyed it.

After I dressed and was ready to leave, I asked him would he give me his false penis as a souvenir.

"Never happen, never happen." He shook his head. "Have several more cities to visit and only one artificial penis."

Just as different ethnic groups have their peculiarities, so do different age groups, and I have observed a consistent pattern with my customers according to their specific age brackets.

The youngest customer I have ever had was seventeen, and

the oldest was seventy-two. However, both these extremes are very rare.

In the old-style brothels of the 1930s and 1940s, I believe there was such a thing as "cherry popping": an occasion when a father would send his adolescent son along to an understanding prostitute for an introduction to sex.

These days, the few youths who visit an establishment like mine come up under their own steam. Nevertheless, these kids are usually very nervous and very quick, and climax almost immediately. They have the strength to climax two or three times, and depending on whether they can afford it or if the prostitute really likes them, they may go again a second time, and maybe a third time, in the same half an hour.

When the men reach their early twenties, they usually come up to my house in groups. At this age they are still a little self-conscious and give each other Dutch courage by the glassful. They are relatively easy to handle and last a little longer than the adolescents.

When men reach their late twenties they have also reached the height of their sexual strength, but far from being desirable as lovers, they are considered by professional girls to be a nuisance. The late twenties are the ones the girls like the least, because they demand every different position in the book, and their snotty attitude is: "I'm young, I'm handsome, I really don't need to use a prostitute, but since I'm here, I will get my money's worth."

By contrast, men in their thirties and forties are the ones the prostitutes like best.

These are the men who know what it's all about. They often go twice in half an hour, and for most girls, it is a pleasure to service them. They usually look after their bodies, work out in a gym, play tennis, and wear nice-smelling colognes and after-shaves. They really appreciate a woman and are not too demanding. The men in their thirties and forties are not too choosy about whether a girl is twenty or thirty, as long as she is attractive and has a nice personality.

Men between forty and fifty are similar in their attitude to the previous group except they usually request a blow job instead of a screw. They are from the generation whose wives are not so liberal about going down on them, so they come to a brothel for what they cannot get at home.

In my experience and opinion, a man has certainly peaked sexually and begun to decline in his late forties.

Men in their fifties start asking for very young girls, prefer-ably Lolita or "daughter" types. These customers are generally wealthy semiretired businessmen who winter in Miami and fly between there, Puerto Rico, Las Vegas, and New York for their pleasure seeking. They usually have a year-round suntan and are true gentlemen, arriving often with a bottle of Scotch or per-fume for the madam. Men over fifty start to feel that what they lack in performance they make up for in generosity. They always seek more privacy than the younger men, are gentle lovers, and can make it only once per hour, if at all.

Such men often seem to go through a kind of "penopause," leaving their wives to go off with some very much younger woman. Indeed, they have created a new market in the business for Lolitas, real or phony. Some twenty-five-year-old girls, with the right dress and makeup, can be passed off as sweet seven-teen. One famous property tycoon complained to his pretty nineteen-year-old daughter that her girlfriends were getting too old for his taste. I always have had a rule not to have minors in a brothel and risk more trouble with the law.

Men over sixty are usually content to give or receive a blow job. Their problem is rarely achieving orgasm, but often it is difficult for them to get a spontaneous hard-on. They practically have to fold their flaccid cocks into a girl and let them sprout into a full erection in the warmth of her vagina. It is a real test of a professional's tact and technique to prevent her man going off "half-cocked."

But it is dangerous to take such sexual senility for granted. A kindly old Philadelphia banker, known to the call girls as Papa Serge because of his gentle, paternal manner, once made a date with me. He took me to a show on Broadway and then gave me a sumptuous meal in a magnificent restaurant. Seated in his limousine on the way back to his suite at the Waldorf, I felt sorry for him. I would have liked to give him a great time, but at his age, he could not fuck his way out of a paper bag.

Or so I thought. We had hardly got through the front door when he had torn off my dress and my panties, and thrown me on the bed. Dropping to his knees, he worked on my clitoris for half an hour with such skill and artistry that I had two superb orgasms. I have never earned my money so easily and so enjoyably. And then he made love to me with a fine, stiff cock; it just took him a little longer than with a younger man, but who was grumbling?

One famous movie magnate, now deceased, fucked well into his seventies. I know because he dated me several times. When he was staying in New York, he called me up and asked me to bring with me another girl, since his seventeen-year-old girlfriend was bisexual. I was more than ready to oblige and brought a very attractive girl to make sure that nobody would be left out. At his penthouse apartment, Mr. Magnate, dressed in a fancy black silk kimono, opened the door to me himself and introduced us to his partner—tall, slim, blond, and very good-looking. Strangely enough, Mr. Magnate never fucked her himself, at least not in my presence. The routine was for the three girls to perform in front of him while he lolled back in his Louis XV chair beside the bed. Occasionally, his robe would fall open and reveal a healthily erect cock. We were licking, sucking, and kissing to our heart's desire, when his girl leaned over me, as I ministered to her pubic triangle, and whispered that I could relax, as she would fake her orgasm for Mr. Magnate's benefit.

I felt this was an insult to my tongue-work. Why waste such masterly technique on a frigid chick? She was a great actress, however, and gave him the works, hurling herself all over the place with all the requisite groans, moans, and hysterical shrieks. But what genuinely set her going was her vibrator, and she worked herself up to a real climax with it, while I had a session with the girl I had brought with me, who truly appreciated my oral talent.

All this time, Mr. Magnate would watch and jerk off. But once his girlfriend had achieved her faked orgasm, he would throw one of the hookers onto the bed and fuck her good and hard, while the vibrator worked overtime on his companion.

Young or old, Afghan or Eskimo, all men who pay for play in a house of pleasure come under the heading of johns, and fit into one of the following categories.

1. **The Easy Chooser.** He comes in horny and in a rush and hardly has the time for a drink. He just wants to get a quick blow job and absolutely no more involvement. No kissing, no holding, no need for faking it on the girl's part. He is in and out in fifteen minutes.

There is a variation on the type of john who wants only a blow job. This one rationalizes that if he does not put his penis inside a vagina he is not being unfaithful to his wife. Strangely enough, this is usually the kind of man who was one of the biggest and wildest playboys before he was married.

2. **The Lover.** He gets emotionally involved with a prostitute, requests her all the time, and doesn't want to see anybody else. He tells her his life story and often wants to convert her—take her away from all this—usually without offering her any alternate means of support. The Lover is happy only if he feels the girl is satisfied with their lovemaking. He is time-consuming but worth the effort, because the Lover is always a steady customer for as long as his love affair lasts. Once a john, always a john!

3. **The Whore-at-Heart.** He likes variety without being especially selective and always prefers the atmosphere of a madam's house to that of a private call girl. He usually brings a bottle of booze or some other gift for the madam, feels very much at home in the brothel, and goes through several girls in the course of a night. By the time he is finished, it is usually approaching dawn, and for the extra fee he often decides to use the pull-out-sofa privileges and sleep over.

4. **The Don Juan.** He comes carrying tales of all the gorgeous airline stewardesses, secretaries, and models he has slept with and who are all after his fantastic body. This type is always young, not necessarily good-looking, and almost never good in bed, either. You often wonder where he gets the strength to spend money at your house, because from the stories he tells, it sounds like he has a pretty good business going for himself!

5. **The Introvert High Roller.** This man, usually more of an intellectual than the average client, wants to see a girl only once in his lifetime and never again. He uses the madams because he knows they have connections with call girls all over the city and can give him access to the variety he craves. He is either a hard-

working bachelor concentrating too hard on his career to hang around parties and pick up girls; or, if he is married, he usually turns up in the summer when his wife is on vacation. He will call any time of the day or night, whenever the urge strikes him.

6. **The Haggler or Bargain Hunter.** He sits down and hangs around for half an hour smoking as many of your cigarettes and drinking as much of your liquor as he can get his hands on while making up his mind whether he will go at all. He puts you out of your way to get a special type of girl, even if there are several already sitting around, and when he finally decides to give it a try, and you are about to straighten out finances, he gives you a hassle and tries to chisel down your prices. He usually throws in how much it cost him to park his car.

7-A. **The Temporary Impotent.** He is impotent on account of too much to drink, fatigue, a nagging wife, tranquilizers, a fall in the stock market, or pressure at the office. But whatever the cause, it is generally short-lived, and when he comes back in another week he will probably be a good, strong lover again. This man is often the slightly nervous, sensitive type. With him we always have patience and try to give him a second chance.

7-B. **The Permanent Impotent.** He likes lots of girls in group scenes or likes to watch lesbian scenes and doesn't care whether the girls are black, white, or green. His permanent debility is caused either by age, illness, such as diabetes, or some massive complex, and his preferences include fingering the girls until they climax (or fake it), just eating them, and trying to masturbate himself while the girl looks on, and some even like being anally penetrated with a dildo or even go as far as carrots, sticks, beads on a string, ice cubes, or any other miscellany that will go up there.

Twelve

Whipped (S)cream!

As the reputation of my house grew, I attracted more and more people with "special requirements"; mostly men but sometimes women. They were hounded as perverts, weirdos, freaks, even maniacs, and psychiatrists and sexologists spoke condescendingly of their aberrations. At first I felt awkward with them, but I soon began to appreciate that they were often people whose intensity of sexual experience enabled them to get real enjoyment far greater than was dreamed of by those straights for whom sex was a bodily function, no more significant than washing their hands. What do we mean by "abnormal sexuality"? Something that does not conform to the banal and simple in-and-out and up-and-down which became accepted in bygone societies of peasants and shepherds? If the sole purpose of sex is procreation, then virtually every embellishment or stroke of fantasy has to be considered a perversion.

And I came into contact with them all. There were the fetishists, who focused their affection on some object: lingerie, shoes, rubber or leather garments, etc. Others were turned on by dirty talk, either actively when making love, or as passive listeners, known in French as *écouteurs*. There were devotees of "the golden shower," who desired nothing more than to be pissed on or sometimes to drink urine. There is an affinity between some homosexuals and urine, as evidenced by the guys who hang around urinals and try to fuck a man who has arrived merely for an innocent pee. One of my most extravagant customers used to lie in a bathtub filled half with champagne and half with urine. The champagne was easy, at a price, but it was an effort to find enough girls with sufficiently full bladders.

I had the exhibitionists, who, like rapists, delighted in the hysterical response of their victims; and at the other extreme, the voyeurs, who got their kicks at being unobserved while they gazed at, for instance, a woman undressing, and in that way resembled the obscene telephone callers, smug in their anonymity. Because of my strict rule against employing minors, I had to decline serving pedophiles.

One of my biggest groups was transvestites, rarely homosexuals and frequently married men with families. They were so fastidious with their clothing and their makeup that they were very time-consuming, but when the metamorphosis had been effected, I would let them mingle with my girls, and sometimes they would even be approached by one of my clients.

Quite often, transvestites were also masochists, and there are probably more misconceptions about sadists and masochists than about any other sexual group. These people play a complex game in which eroticism is indissolubly fused with the giving or receiving of pain, and after my experience with Carl, I had become something of a specialist in S/M. I discovered within myself both sadistic and masochistic tendencies, but what fascinates me is the mental dimension to these games. A rich department-store owner would come to my house, where he was known as "our humble servant," in order to wear a sex apron and walk around with a broom and dustpan and clean up after the girls, wash their bras and panties, and do the dishes. And he was not unique. Some of America's wealthiest and most influential businessmen make the pilgrimage to be whipped, beaten, dressed as a girl, tied down, or chained to a bed. They pay well, and I serve them with the greatest of pleasure. These men appreciate a harsh, dominant woman, usually with long blond or raven-black hair, not necessarily very young or very beautiful, but willing to participate fully in their theater of cruelty, whether the scenario be a harmless trifle or a passionate epic.

One particularly bizarre episode stands out in my memory. I was at home one evening when I was called up by Laura, who asked me to accompany her to a very special party for which I would be paid handsomely. She referred to her clients as Mr. and Mrs. Showbiz, and they lived in an old brownstone in Manhattan. But she confided their true identities to me: one of the country's most successful film producers and his wife, whom he referred to always as Anna, a beautiful British actress who had established an outstanding reputation on the classical stage on both sides of the Atlantic.

I am not one of those people who fawn over celebrities and are overawed by the jet set, but I must admit that I was looking forward eagerly to meeting this couple. However, when our host opened the door, I recognized that he had visited my establishment a few months previously and had asked me to provide him with a couple of fifteen-year-old Lolitas, which I had refused.

There had been stories in magazines of wild swinging parties and cocaine, and the house certainly had an opulence which would have provided the perfect setting. Mr. Showbiz strutted around, quite the lord and master, but as Laura showed me around while we waited for Anna to get ready, she told me that it was his wife who paid for everything.

Anna had prepared a rich, soapy bubble bath for us in their big, heart-shaped tub. Laura and I slowly and seductively undressed each other and stepped into the water, where we continued to caress our bodies and rub the soap into our skin. Laura leaned over me, her firm nipples brushing my neck as she seized the showerhead and trained a jet of warm, tingling water over my clitoris. It was bliss, and I took one of her feet and lovingly soaped, rinsed, and sucked each of her toes. Under the play of the water, I reached my first orgasm, and then Laura spread her legs invitingly. How I adored that fabulous, purple pussy! I savored her labial lips, thick and meaty, and I felt her clitoris swelling in my mouth while I cupped her strong buttocks in my hands, thrusting her body harder against my face and my tongue ever deeper within her.

All this time, Mr. and Mrs. Showbiz were watching us attentively from the doorway. Anna moaned softly; she had been masturbating herself against the soft silk of her gown. Her quivering orgasm and her husband's murmured incitements spurred Laura and me to yet more frantic activity, and when Anna joined us in the tub, everybody seemed to be kissing everywhere. There were tongues in my ears, on my cheeks, my lips, my hair, even fluttering over my eyes. At last, Anna asked us to come into the bedroom.

The king-size bed was surrounded by velvet wallpaper and floor-to-ceiling mirrors. Laura had been there before and knew exactly what was demanded of us. To my amazement, she tore off the gown which Anna had put on after drying her body, and threw her roughly onto the bed. It was my first experience with a female masochist, and it was a shock to see that porcelain-fine skin being scratched, her shapely limbs bruised, and the ripe globes of her breasts being savagely bitten by Laura, who had been transformed into a raging Fury. Laura thrust some silk shawls into my hand and ordered me to tie Anna's feet to the bed. Then her husband gave me a double-headed dildo. I smeared some Vaseline on it and drove the monstrous tool into her dripping cunt.

"Shove the other end up her ass, hard and fast," Laura whispered.

So while I attended to the lower half of her body, Laura slapped her face and punched her breasts, and all the time Anna's face registered agony and pleasure, but I think that I was the only one who was not turned on by her bestial whimpering. Mr. Showbiz had a lecherous expression as he watched. He treated himself to several poppers and lines of cocaine which he had spread upon a mirror. Every now and then, he halted us to give Anna a chance to take a sniff of the white powder, and eventually Laura told me to stop working her over with the dildo. But there was no letup for Anna. Laura stuffed two high-speed vibrators into her pussy and her ass. Her passion mounted to a frenzy until Mr. Showbiz had the buzzing machines removed, dropped his purple pajama pants and mounted her. They fucked like wild animals, and as they reached their peak, Anna was still screaming how wonderful it was and begging for more.

I felt something like anger. Anna was such a beautiful woman, and if we had been alone I could have shown her so much tenderness. Punishment, however, was what she wanted, what she paid for, and what she got. But I did tell Laura not to call me again for a return visit.

The scene left a lingering impression on me, and I figured maybe the actress needed the debasing to balance the heavy adulation she gets from her theater audiences and movie fans.

Who knows? All *I* know is she's lucky she earns so much, because she spends big money on prostitutes. Laura alone is paid $1,500 to stop by five times a week and give a convincing performance.

Abraham is another case who needs to be cruelly degraded before he can get his rocks off. He is a wealthy forty-five-year-old Jewish businessman who got his first taste of sex under the most extreme kind of conditions as a teenage prisoner in a Nazi concentration camp.

A tough woman guard, naked under her raincoat, ordered him behind the lavatories one night and forced him to perform cunnilingus. To this day Abraham remembers vividly the fear mixed with reluctant excitement that he felt. And he has failed to overcome the trauma to the extent that he cannot have sex without re-creating the sights, sounds, and smells of that carnal moment.

I came in contact with Abraham when he called the house where I worked before I became a madam, requesting a girl who spoke fluent German, was reasonably strongly built, and could order him about. The madam assured him I was tailor-made for the part and sent me to his apartment in a luxury high-rise building in the East Fifties.

Abraham, after greeting me politely at the door, wanted to get right down to brass tacks, and the first thing he did was lead me to a locked hall closet.

The slight, pale man fumbled with the locks, and from the way he acted, I thought he must be hiding the crown jewels. But as he pulled open the door with a grand gesture, I saw that the closet contained nothing else but six or seven original SS rain-coats—and the smell of decaying rubber was so thick inside you could cut it with a knife.

This man begged me to undress and put the raincoat on over my naked body and carry out a mock SS raid and a beating.

"Don't forget to put on the belt," he reminded me as he attached a swastika to the arm and handed me a toy gun.

The scene was to proceed with me going out of the bedroom while he arranged himself, naked, on the bed with his head toward the closed door.

Outside the door, I had to bang with my fists—*Boom! Boom! Boom*—and roar out in German: "Gestapo here! Open the door immediately!"

But there is no reply. So I kick the door open and burst in, to find him lying there with his penis in his hand. "*Herr* Cohen," I demand in a menacing voice.

"No, no, I'm Mr. Smith," he says meekly, pretending to tremble.

"Don't lie to me, you're a Jew—*Verdammter Jude, Schwein-hund*." *Bam! bam!* I slam him across the face.

Little Abraham quivers all over, gets an instant erection, and is very excited. He starts waffling about the "bloody Jews" and how he hopes every last one of them gets what he deserves.

"Shut up, Jew!" I hiss, and to assure that he obeys, I sit on his face and force him to eat me. Then I get mad because he does it wrong, and take off my belt and spank him until he is almost about to climax. Just then he calls a halt to activity.

"Let's stop and do it all again," he pleads. So we repeat the scene once again. The *third* time, while I spank him hard, Abraham jerks off.

The poor man is happy and pleased to pay me, but this kind of thing also makes me sad, because I'm half Jewish, and even though I was only a baby during World War II, I hate to be confronted with things like this.

Still another man who got his hang-up in a war camp is the rabbi who can make it only with non-Jewish girls, and only after they paint him all over with swastikas.

These sexually unorthodox not only have their favorite scene, they also have their favorite atmosphere and conditions. For instance, full moons and gloomy or stormy weather are often highly stimulating. I often think they are as predictable as the little blue boy in those miniature European weather vanes. When the weather is lousy, out they come. Perhaps people who dig suffering at any time consider it an added bonus when the weather is mean to them, too. Masochists are also very intrigued by umbrellas, which represent to them a potential weapon of chastisement.

Umbrellas are so important to those who love to suffer that the biggest S/M supply store in Manhattan is a West Side umbrella shop where I purchased most of the contents of my "goodie bag."

Every good master needs at the very minimum a good set of manacles, whips, rawhides, handcuffs, chains, paddles, and a dildo. Those who specialize exclusively in the S/M scene have much more variety and perhaps more expensive, subtler instruments. I have one lovely slave who combs Europe searching for medieval leg irons and handcuffs, and he always brings his own bondage accessories for his special scenes.

Incidentally, this man recently visited my fellow country-woman, Monique van Cleef—a madam who ran a famous house of pain in New Jersey until she was raided, and is now experimenting in The Hague with a brand-new treat for masochists called cell isolation. In her house this woman has had a special cell built in which she locks her customers after she has clapped them in irons. Sometimes she strings their hands to the ceiling. I understand she is doing a roaring business.

A young slave customer of mine named Nicky took me to the umbrella store one gloomy day to equip himself for my slave scenes. Jonny Starr, the Negro manager of the store, who has since worked for me as a stud, slave, and master, showed me his collection of whips and paddles, all of which I tested out against my hand or Nicky's ass. As I was making my choice, I happened to glance at the store window, and standing there was a well-dressed man completely mesmerized.

Even through the glass I could recognize that familiar spaniel look they all have of "Beat me, hit me, please."

In order to tease him, I gave Nicky another smack on his ass, and the whip made a swishing noise that made this window-shopper get all shook up.

Then I got the bright idea that if I was investing so much money in the new instruments of bondage and torture, I should assure myself of at least one customer, so I walked outside and stood alongside him pretending to study the umbrella display.

I happened to be dressed appropriately that day, with black leather pants, black turtleneck sweater, high boots, and my hair in a severe upswept style. The combination of me and the man-acles drove him to speak to me.

"You handle that whip so beautifully," he said in Hungarianaccented English. "I bet you could do a lot with it to make people happy."

"If you think I could make you happy, please allow me to try," I answered.

"That I would just love." He glowed. "Where can I find you, and when will I come?"

"Come at six P.M. sharp," I ordered, because with slaves there is never an approximate time. They are always punctual because of the need to be obedient. I handed him my card, and he nodded and walked away.

As expected, the window-shopper arrived at the stroke of six, all sad-eyed and full of expectancy. That night I tried out everything in my new goodie bag, which he loved so much he became a regular slave until he moved away from New York a year and a half later.

A masochist, no matter how he was first acquired, usually becomes a faithful one-master or -mistress slave.

My ability to spot a masochist is uncanny. I can recognize a slave in any environment, and often before he knows it himself, because I can read eyes the way palmists read hands.

This happened on the beach in Puerto Rico with a famous New York City disc jockey I'll call William H. Levy. The man definitely had a masochistic tendency but had never acknowledged it, probably out of fear that the reality might either disgust or addict him. Levy was wearing dark glasses when we were introduced, and as we stood talking at the water's edge, I could feel those strange vibrations, so I asked him to remove the shades.

"I want to see your eyes, because in the eyes of a human being lies his soul," I told him.

He unsuspectingly took off his sunglasses, and straight away I said, "I bet you're a masochist."

The disc jockey's reaction was startling. I had really hit a nerve. His whole casual attitude changed, and I could tell he was suddenly afraid of me.

To win back his confidence, I told him that I was a professional with a knack for the S/M scene. I even made him confess something he had never told anyone in his life, including—and especially—his nice wife.

For years he has had a recurring dream, and he starts the story this way: "As I get off the air, I see myself dialing the telephone number of a woman in black, whose face I can't see, but she has a mane of black hair.

"She orders me to come to her, but just as she is about to tell me where and when, the phone falls from my hand, and when I try to call her, my finger always slips from the dial. She will be furious with me, thinking that I am playing games, and when I hurry to her house, I know that I am hours late and deserve to be punished.

"She is seated in a high chair at the other end of a room, and she orders me to crawl to her on my hands and knees. But when I try to do so, the floor is somehow turned into a kind of conveyer belt, running in the opposite direction, so that the more I scramble toward her, the farther away she is. I am obsessed by her, and my knees are bruised by my frantic efforts to reach her. At last, I struggle to her feet, but she is on the phone and ignores me. She is making strange clicking and whirring noises, and these drive me crazy with jealousy. I stretch out a hand and touch her, but she kicks me hard in the face with her spiked heel. Then she laughs at me, hurls obscenities, and spits at me. Standing erect, she orders me to lick her shoes. Then I am chained and manacled before her, and she is brandishing a huge bull whip, which she cracks menacingly above my head. Finally, she does whip me until the blood is streaming from my back and face and then, throwing the whip aside, rips my clothes off with her long scarlet nails with which she tears my throat until it too is dripping blood."

Levy and I were staying in the same hotel, and in the middle of the afternoon my phone rang. He wanted to know if I had thought about his problem.

"Yes, I have," I said, and started spinning him a long fantasy over the phone of how he would get shipwrecked and rescued by naked islanders—only to discover too late they were cannibals who would cook him and eat him.

I could tell the story was turning him on as his heavy breathing came through the phone. "Hang up and come straight to my room," I ordered him, just like the woman in black.

He arrived wearing only his bathrobe and was at such a pitch that all I had to do was spank him lightly with my hand on his thigh, and he climaxed.

The world of make-believe is so delicate and sensitive that the essential mood can be shattered by the least lapse in reality. Therefore, the fantasy you spin, the clothes you wear, and the atmosphere you create are absolutely important.

Early in my career as a practicing mistress, I welcomed to my house a man who called himself Marco Polo, who was in fact a famous public personage who makes TV appearances all over the world and regularly has his picture in *Time* magazine.

When this man walked into my living room, I was looking very feminine, wearing a diaphanous nightgown, my hair hanging demurely to my shoulders. "You're not the type of woman I expected to see," he said, backing off. "You couldn't scare me."

"Perhaps if you will be patient for a little while, I could find you a woman who could," I said, and as he made himself comfortable in the armchair, I faded into the bedroom and came back wearing a black leather outfit, with fishnet stockings, and my hair in a severe pulled-back style. My face was made up to fit the role, and I lowered my voice.

The transformation was perfect for him, and immediately he was reassured. For half an hour we sat in the living room discussing what was his hang-up—and our plan to satisfy it. Marco Polo described to me a set of symptoms that were familiar with many successful and powerful men.

As absolute ruler in his corporation, he manipulates the men beneath him like a puppeteer. However, this daytime domineering makes him feel insecure, and as a balance to reality, he craves being submissive. These powerful men become slaves to release the tension of running other people's lives.

Having recognized Marco Polo's preference, I suggested the bedroom, which was prepared with flickering candles and black lights to create a spooky atmosphere, and once inside, his uptight living-room manner disappeared; instead, he lived out his fantasy.

Marco Polo's desire is to make you believe he is some kind of docile animal, and he needs first to be talked into a different world—which is the mentally exhausting part of it. It can take more than an hour, gradually and convincingly getting him into his fantasy while dressing him with wigs, makeup, handcuffs, and leg irons. I then add a blindfold, which is often done to increase the thrill of an unknown fear and humiliation. To masochists, the feeling of being in bondage and blindfolded as well can be compared to the classic double ecstasy.

While he lies blindfolded, bound, and helpless, I talk about the hidden secrets of the ocean, the storm-tossed breakers, crowned by frothing white foam, the fishermen fighting the sea to cast their nets into the depths, and the beautiful mermaid whom they long to catch. One of my assistants, Mary Lou, comes into the room, and together we place him on the bed, with his head at the foot. Binding his legs together in bandages so that he now has a tail, we tell him that he is our mermaid, and we throw a net over him.

I take off my clothes and poise my body above his face, inviting him to eat me, but only letting him feel the touch of my pubic hair against his mouth, and trying to sniff his way to my cunt. Whenever he gets near to achieving what he so much desires, I pull back and tease him till he is frantic.

Now is the time for our mystery guest, Jonny, the black umbrella salesman. Marco Polo would never admit to homosexuality; that is a taboo which cannot be broken. Or can it? He has just enough slack in his chains to be able to play with my tits, and I allow him the pleasure of licking my pussy. At a sign from me, Jonny silently climbs behind me and slides his enormous cock between my legs. Marco Polo, amazed and unseeing, finds that this magic woman has mysteriously grown a penis, and how he loves it! I order him to suck *my* cock, and while he is doing so, I climb off Jonny and leave the two of them together. We free Marco Polo's hands so that he can jerk off. When Jonny eventually shoots his load into his mouth, Marco Polo comes with a loud groan all over his own belly. Only after Jonny has slipped away, as soundlessly as he came, do we remove Marco Polo's blindfold.

A session like this takes plenty of time, during which I cannot take phone calls or receive other guests, so it has to cost a minimum of $1,000.

Clothes make the man, and also the scene.

I have an entire wardrobe for transvestites and fetishists, including special nighties, lace and leather dresses, garter belts, stockings, big-size padded bras and girdles, gloves, and oversize women's high heels.

At the time I was going seriously into the different-sex trade, I went to a small shop on Lexington Avenue to buy the appropriate clothes. Being relatively new to the scene, I needed a little guidance, so I walked over to the young gay salesman. "Can I help you?" he asked, and all of a sudden I could see *those eyes*.

"Yes, you can help me," I replied. "You see, I need a wardrobe for transvestites, and you look to me like you know what it's all about."

At first his mouth fell open, but then he smiled. "Well, dear, now that you put it that way, let me suggest to you these divine garter belts, these darling black crotchless panties," he lisped effeminately, "and how about something in a fishnet stocking?" The sales assistant also recommended a few sexy nighties, in case one of my slaves was in the right mood to wear them.

The first night I had the new collection, I had a fetishist who was so thrilled I could dress him in such heavenly clothes he almost came by looking at them.

Snapping my fingers and slapping my hands together like a bossy mother teaching her school-age son to dress, I ordered him into them. But he was so enchanted being in the new bra and panties that he climaxed before he got the nightdress on.

This man doesn't take more than half an hour usually: to make sure he got something more for his money, I gave him a friendly spanking as a dessert.

Transvestites and masochists will perform the most incredible kinds of emotional and physical acts in their pursuits of gratification, but basically they never fuck. They come by masturbating or having it done to them, or with a dildo in their anus, or, like the one I just mentioned, with no help at all. Or in some cases, they are not allowed to come at all.

One of my nicest and most faithful slaves was Tame Timmy, a professional gigolo. Coming from an aristocratic English family, he was sent to a famous public school, where he was regularly beaten and flogged. When he arrived in America, he patronized the racetracks and casinos, where he met many wealthy, older women. As he was handsome and cultured and endowed with an upper-class scorn of work, he was able to find ladies who would keep him in opulent idleness; indeed, four of them went so far as to marry him.

When I met him, he was enjoying his third divorce, from which he was the one who received the alimony, but I was something special for him. With me he could play his favorite role: that of submissive slave, and he was the one who paid. As he was between marriages, instead of coming to my house, he invited me to his place. I arrived to find him totally engrossed in a horror movie on TV. He wanted his session with me, but he could not tear himself away from the film so, after first dressing him in girls' clothes, I took a long rope and lashed him to the bed from which he could watch the screen. I made sure that the knots were good and tight and even tied up his penis and scrotum with surgical wire so that he looked like a gift-wrapped sausage. Then I went out.

An hour later, I returned. Boris Karloff was still doing his stuff, but Timmy was in a frightful state. He was bursting for a pee, and his penis had gone a delicate shade of purple. But I was deaf to his pleading and busied myself lighting candles. Instead of letting him go to the bathroom, I made him crawl around the icy floor of the kitchen, which further increased the pressure on his bladder. I climbed on his back and rode him around the apartment, whacking the fine, round ass of my steed, and jerking the rope tied around his throat to rein him in. Only then did I undo his penis—since I did not want the restriction of his blood flow to permanently disable him. While the movie flickered eerily, I dripped hot wax from the candles onto his balls and cock, and he screamed in agony. And to cap everything, I made him fuck me with his bladder about to explode. His eyes were popping out of his head with excitement, and we came together in a wild orgasm. At last I led him to the toilet, where I held his penis while he peed like a horse.

Not all S and Ms are harmless or docile, and I heard that when the New York S/M group held a convention this year in a Manhattan hotel, two slaves were so savagely beaten during a demonstration by overenthusiastic masters that they had to be hospitalized.

There are those like the Cucumber Kid, who come to my house wanting all kinds of damage done to them.

This man, who had just been released from the hospital after another girl shoved a cucumber up his ass and split him in a dozen pieces, wants you to impale him on a hat pin, drip hot wax on his balls, or do anything else that will cause him unbearable pain.

The kind of treatment that the Cucumber Kid wanted does more than cause pain, and I refuse to do anything that might cause anyone real damage, although I myself was almost murdered in my own house in a freak scene gone haywire.

It began innocently enough when a man named Larry Lerner called up late one night with a referral from Madeleine Henry, and he wanted to come by. I vaguely remembered Madeleine referring to him once as a bit unusual and strange, particularly when he was drunk. I honestly didn't feel like any more business, because it was 3:00 A.M. I had shut up shop and was relaxing over a fruit juice with a girl named Sarah, my roommate and also a working girl. But I had promised Madeleine I would take good care of her customers, and to stick to my word, I let him come up.

Lerner was drunk as a skunk when he arrived, and at once I regretted letting him come. If I'd had my radar working properly, I would have realized he was trouble and told him to come back tomorrow. I hate drunks at anytime, let alone at three in the morning.

They are slow in their sexual activity, and altogether they are a pain in the neck. I figured normal sex would be impossible with Lerner, but I couldn't quite figure the man's number. There was something kind of sinister about his eyes. They were alternately harsh and dreamy. As I've said, I usually can tell a lot by a man's eyes, but this night I really got the signals crossed. I decided he was a masochist.

"Why don't we do something different?" I suggested. "You are going to be my slave, and I'm going to be your master, and I want you to do exactly what I say."

"No," he said, "I'm gonna be the sadist."

"Maybe you did not understand me. We are going to reverse the roles. In this house, you are the slave and I am the boss. If you don't like it, you can fuck off right now."

I was taking a chance with this attractive young man. But he smiled, poured himself a Scotch, and paid up front a couple of hundred dollars.

I decided to use the living room and pushed the nearby furniture to one side while he undressed. Then I got out my goodie bag and put him in bondage with rawhide ties, handcuffs, and a gag. I also put him in a blindfold, but I did it all very gently and did not beat him at all.

We laid him down in the middle of the floor while Sarah sat

swiveling herself in the chair, teasing him and saying how ridiculous he looked.

During the fifteen or twenty minutes, Lerner showed little life and was altogether a very boring slave, so in order to hurry this thing along I whispered to Sarah I was going to the kitchen to get some amyl nitrate to speed him up a bit.

And this reckless gesture was the worst thing I could have done, but I was then naive about the lethal combination of alcohol and drugs.

Immediately after I popped the amyl nitrate under his nose, he stiffened. "What is that you're giving me?" he choked.

"I'm just giving you a harmless popper," I told him, "so don't worry about it. Inhale, inhale."

But Lerner was momentarily panicked. "Everything has gone completely black!" he bellowed. "Get me out of here!"

"It can't last more than thirty seconds," I assured him, but he was impossible to placate. So Sarah and I spent the next ten minutes removing the blindfold and the bonds, by which time we supposed he had calmed down and was over his experience.

But we couldn't have been more wrong.

As he reached toward me on the pretext of getting a cigarette from the coffee table, I saw the sadistic look in his eyes too late. Before I could jump out of the way, his huge hamfist had landed a vicious blow to my jaw and sent me reeling.

The madman pounced on me, grabbed my long hair, and started hammering violently at the back of my neck, my chest, and my groin. He had gone stark mad, berserk.

Sarah was screaming and made a few attempts to pull him off me, but he sent her running with a karate blow to the head. She vanished, and I didn't know where, because I was too busy trying to save my skin.

The savage beating went on for about fifteen minutes, blood was coming from my nose and lips, and it was a wonder I was not already dead. Any other woman would have crumpled already, but luckily I have a really hard head.

To show you how hard it is, once I was riding my bicycle along the canal in Holland when the car in front braked suddenly and threw me forward onto its roof, then down to the ground. When I stood up and felt my head, it was a little bit sore, but no bruises. There was a big, deep hole in the car.

After what seemed an eternity, the telephone mercifully rang, and I grabbed it, and Sarah was at the other end, saying, "Hang in there, Xaviera, I'm coming up with the police." This to me was the worst thing she could do, because you don't call the police up to a whorehouse! But on the other hand, to just let me get killed was no good, either.

At that point Lerner said: "I'm going to kill you." And with murder in his eyes he picked up the heavy wooden coffee table and held it over my head.

Just then the door opened, and Lerner dropped the table, which missed me by a hairbreadth. But he still had hold of what was left of my hair and was still threatening to kill me, although he was rational enough to try to put on his underpants with the other hand.

I seized the opportunity to struggle out of his grasp, and I was never so relieved to see a policeman in my life.

"What seems to be the trouble?" the two fresh-faced young cops asked. As if they couldn't see for themselves! My eyes were as big as artichokes, my nose was bleeding like a tap, and my mouth was three times its normal size. I looked like I'd gone five rounds with Muhammad Ali.

"Oh, nothing much, officers," I said. "Just a little family

squabble. You know, my boyfriend here had a little too much to drink and got a bit frisky."

If that looked like a family squabble, my name must be Father Christmas, because on the floor in full view were my whips, manacles, and handcuffs all around.

I tried to bend over to pick them up, but the pain in my body made it impossible. Sarah could see what I was trying to do, so she scooped up the stuff and put it in a closet.

"Do you want to press charges, then?" the cops asked.

How could I press charges against a client? I could be hung by the heels from the Empire State Building and not be able to press charges in the business I'm in.

"No, thank you, gentlemen, but if I could ask you to escort him off the premises, I would be very grateful."

When the police left and the shock wore off, I really felt sorry for myself. My hair was falling out in big handfuls, a tooth was chipped, the guy had banged me black and blue in my vagina, and my stomach felt like I just gave birth to a dinosaur. I had a terrible headache, probably minor brain concussion.

So far I had kept my cool, but by now I was at breaking point, and I needed a strong shoulder, so I called my boyfriend. Half an hour later he came over and took me to the emergency room at the hospital on Seventy-second and York.

After what I went through there, it was a toss-up whether I might have been better just staying at home. We sat there waiting for half an hour before anybody even bothered to see what was wrong. Then someone came along and asked a whole lot of questions: name, address, education, previous illnesses, whether I had ever been there before, and if so, did I pay my bill.

After about another hour a doctor came by and knocked me

on my knee, knocked me on my head, knocked me on my back and said: "X rays."

I was directed into a room where this X-ray technician with a black moustache told me to get into a paper robe that opens down the front, and climb onto the table. He watched me undress, and he could hardly believe his eyes when he saw how badly I was beaten.

"My God, whatever happened to you?" he asked.

To hell with it, I thought, I might as well tell him the truth in twenty words, no more, and I could use a little sympathy.

"Ah, you know, an innocent S/M scene. It got out of hand."

But sympathy is not what I got. As I glanced out of the corner of my swollen eye, I could see there was a hard-on in his pants. "Before we start," he said with a slimy smile, "how about a blow job?"

With all I'd gone through, all I needed was a horny X-ray technician at five in the morning! "Baby, get your work done; one animal a night is enough."

"If you give me a blow job I'll give you the X rays free; otherwise it will cost you $150," he persisted.

If I could have conjured up the strength, I would have kicked him in the balls. As it was, all I could do was to mumble, "Forget about it, Charley, quit, split, get on with your work and send me the bill."

The technician was crushed but not completely discouraged. "All right," he said. "But can you let me have your card?"

Thirteen

An Adult Tale,
or, Fantasy and Me

"**9** am a four-times married contessa, simply rolling in money left me by my three husbands, who have all mysteriously died," I tell the man sitting fully dressed in my living room.

"My fourth husband is ailing and may not survive the night . . ."

"Yes, yes, go on, go on," he urges impatiently in his thin, piping voice. "What happened to these men? Tell me!"

"The first, poor man, drowned right before my eyes in the sea at Deauville. I, uh, sort of held his head under water.

"The second, rest his soul, died an agonizing death when his bedroom caught fire, and I could not get the door open to let him out."

"The third?" he prods. "What happened to him?"

"It was in Switzerland, not long ago. I was admiring a fabulous view. He fell off a mountain—clumsy!"

While I am spinning the story, the man sits there spell-bound. His bony hand, shaking from the first stages of Parkinson's disease, goes to his pants pocket and starts tampering with his cock.

H. Christian Andersen, as he likes to be called, is the scion of one of America's wealthiest shipping families. He is also one of the biggest-spending eccentrics I have ever met.

People like him prefer much more exotic and ingenious humiliation than the usual masochist. They will pay any amount; sometimes, the more you charge, the happier they are; and some of their scenes would bend your brain.

H. Christian Andersen doesn't want sex, and he pretends you're a rich but chiseling woman. In other words, he comes to a brothel for a different kind of tail—a fantasy tale. An imaginative storyteller, which I can claim to be, can earn a really fat fee from this kind of client by spinning out the episodes over a series of days.

"What about your present husband?" Andersen demands to know. "What's bothering him?"

"Poor man," I say, "the doctor thinks he ate poisoned caviar. He is in terrible agony and may not last the night, but I'll let you know what happened when you come back tomorrow."

He is happy to treat me generously for that little half-hour story, makes his appointment for the following day, and leaves.

I always try my best to give H. Christian Andersen original fairy tales for his money, but if I am distracted and can't invent one sufficiently intriguing, he will sometimes settle for his old favorite, which is my version of *The Emperor's New Clothes*.

In this story I play the role of the *vendeuse*, or saleswoman, at Dior's New York salon, and Andersen takes the part of Mrs. Rich Bitch ordering her new fall wardrobe.

On the first day, we discuss fabrics and inevitably decide the entire collection will be done in crushed velvet—he adores crushed velvet—and satin. That being established, he pays far more than the standard fees for the consultation, out of which I have to buy the fabrics also. Before he comes back the next afternoon, I send out for ten dollars' worth of two fabrics, which he sits and fondles while we plan how we'll make them up.

"Would you prefer to send the fabrics to Paris to be made by Cardin or Dior, or shall we summon one of the couturiers here?" I ask my client. Dior has been dead for several years, but he doesn't know that.

"Bring Dior," he commands.

"These people don't come cheap," I warn him. "Christian Dior will want at least $700 to cross the Atlantic."

"Money is no problem, bring the man here," he repeats, and produces his wallet.

Next day when he comes around to meet with Dior, I have a very sad story to tell him. Dior's plane has been grounded on the polar route in Anchorage, Alaska. "He is stranded in a snowstorm, and the cables, limousines, and hotel bills are mounting," I have to inform him. Naturally, he covers the cost of all that.

While we're waiting for the couturier to arrive, I make the suggestion that his new clothes would fit better if he had some silicone shots to plump up his breasts. "That *is* a splendid idea," he beams babyishly, and pays for a jab on each side of his chest with an empty syringe.

Eventually the clothes are ready, obviously not made by Dior. I had found a gorgeous velvet gown which suited him perfectly, and I drape the finery around him and assure him he is a vision of sartorial splendor. He settles up his massive account, thanks me profusely, and goes merrily on his way. Andersen's non-clothes have cost him dearly, but he is thrilled to pay, and always eager for more tall tales. However, the man has often exhausted my imagination.

Occasionally I feel like telling him: "Hey, H. Christian, I'm running out of stories. Are you sure you don't want to get laid?" I really would like to see him get more value for his money, but he prefers to be taken for a ride.

In fact, one time I really took him for a weird ride, literally. He wanted me to kidnap him!

What's more, he offered such a big ransom for his kidnapping that I could not refuse. Together with a limousine driver I know, I planned to pick Andersen up outside a Fourteenth Street subway station, where he agreed to wait for us with a flower in his buttonhole and a rolled-up newspaper in his hand at twelve noon.

But, seeing he likes to suffer, I kept him waiting till two-thirty, when I pulled up in the black limousine, lured him into the backseat, and stuffed a plastic bag over his head.

We drove him to an upstate motel, where the limo driver kept guard over him for two days, refusing him anything but an occasional paper cup of water and a crust of bread. He was tied to a chair and made to sleep in a straitjacket. On the third day we released him, and he was so delighted with his kidnapping that he paid us a tip on top of the generous ransom money.

Sadomasochists often use props, but rarely, unlike the latter, are they instruments of bondage or torture. It is more often something relatively harmless like some surgical tubing knotted around the private parts, cigarette smoke, or expensive silk scarves.

One client pays me to tie a nautical slipknot around his penis and balls, lead him around the room like a puppy, manipulate it while he sits on the floor and I sit on the bed, and when I want him to climax, I give it a sudden jerk, the knot comes away, and he pops his cookies.

Another john simply wants me to sit in a chair while he sits naked facing me in another chair, and I have to puff on a cigarette and blow the smoke in his face while he plays with himself.

Expensive silk scarves are the hang-up of the president of one of Europe's largest automobile manufacturing companies, whom I will identify as Mr. Bigwheel.

I acquired Mr. Bigwheel as a customer from Madeleine, who used to make lots of money selling him cocaine at highly inflated prices, which he then used in his nocturnal charades.

Mr. Bigwheel's pet scene is having hookers come to his Waldorf Towers suite—always in pairs—to do nothing but stand motionless in front of a three-way mirror while he dances around draping them in Hermés scarves.

When this man is in town, I usually do the first shift myself because I know that before the night is over he will request a whole gaggle of girls, and one previous time I couldn't find enough.

When we arrive at his suite, he greets us wearing a pair of chic silk pajamas and does not attempt to disrobe or expose his body at all during the next two hours, which is how long it generally lasts. However, the hired girls have to undress and put on heavy woolen socks, get back into their own high-heeled shoes, and stand motionless while he does his decorating.

Then he dips cocaine on our breasts and pussycats and eats or sniffs it off and starts going berserk, babbling away in an incoherent mixture of French and Italian.

It becomes very tiring for the girls because, except for the five minutes when we are allowed to lie down while he admires his handiwork, we are on our feet all the time, and those thick woolen socks really make our shoes pinch.

After two uncomfortable but entirely platonic hours, he pays us $200 each, and we dress and leave.

Mr. Bigwheel always keeps me awake throughout the night finding sets of prostitutes to send over to him, and about nine in the morning, when you would think he would be exhausted from all the cocaine and cavorting, he calls up, wants me to come over to straight screw him, boom, boom, ten minutes, in, up, and out. Then he orders breakfast, bathes, and goes off to a business conference, and that night he freaks out in the same fashion all over again.

Another thing that goes over big with some men who want to do anything but screw is wrestling. The Referee, a New York literary critic, has this activity down to a fine art.

The Referee comes to my house carrying a little black case from which he pulls out an old-fashioned flowered garter-belt-corset–type garment. I have to undress in front of him and get into the corset. He loves to see women's flesh bulge out of the tight harness.

Then I have to put on fishnet stockings, crotchless panties and high heels, and lie down on my bed. The Referee undresses, too, and gets on the bed beside me with his black bag.

He opens the treasured bag again and pulls out a neat folder, which I first thought would be the same old pictures of men sucking women and women sucking men, but no, instead it's a whole collection of women wrestlers, which he spreads around the bed.

The pictures are ancient, the paper is yellow, and even though he has looked at them hundreds of times, he still gets juiced up showing them to me. "Look how this one's tits stick up, and look how this one's got her cunt in the air!"

He gets very carried away as we discuss the wrestling postures of the fierce-looking women with their old-fashioned hair styles and muscular bodies.

After a while he puts them all neatly away and takes out another folder full of pictures of movie stars such as Sophia Loren, Gina Lollobrigida, and Brigitte Bardot, as well as beautiful models in ads, and the women all have one thing in common; they are all wearing some kind of foundation garment, like corsets, sexy brassieres, garters, or stockings.

Then the Referee wants me to match them together as wrestling partners. "Who do you think could really give it to the other one?" he asks lasciviously. Apparently I do an expert job of pairing them, because he gets so excited he starts jumping around on the bed and asks me if I have ever wrestled with a woman.

To such people, psychology is one of the most important attributes, so I tell him, "I love to wrestle, and I always win because I am very aggressive." I make up a vivid story about having a fight on the beach in Puerto Rico with a stuck-up English girl with red hair and freckles, whom I couldn't stand on account of some boyfriend.

"Wrestling is my favorite pastime," I boasted, "and I always win, because I am tough. This girl, I grabbed her long hair and swiped her round her face. As she staggered back, I ripped the clothes off her body until all she wore was a garter belt and tattered stockings. She had fine, strong thighs, and I had seized the elastic of her panties in my teeth and torn them to shreds. I raised great welts on her body with my long nails and ended by grasping her juicy pussy and tearing out handfuls of her thick, crisp pubic hair. She fled, screaming in fury."

I could see that as he listened to my story, he got an enormous erection and he sat, jerking off on the side of the bed. I told him how I had gathered a male audience who was cheering me on, and as I narrated my moment of triumph, he came with a puffing and groaning, as if he were the one who was in pain.

Then he got up, washed, dressed, put his pictures back in his bag, paid me a large wad of bills, and left the house without saying another word.

I'm a big hit with the wrestling fanatics because I am strong and sometimes can put on a vicious, dominant act. And that's my problem, because this fatiguing guy, Gorgeous George, will wrestle with nobody but me.

I met Gorgeous George before I was a busy madam and could devote the time it took to tumble around the floor with him, but these days his hang-up is far too time-consuming—and painful—for me.

Gorgeous George is skinny and wiry and rather ugly, but a fabulous conversationalist, a brilliant pianist-composer, a financial wizard, and an accomplished tennis player.

He is also the father of a young son, which amazed me when I found out, because all he ever does for his $150 is roll around the floor and wrestle. He never screws, and he never even jerks off. How, I wondered for a long time, did this man make a baby when he never even climaxes? Then I accidentally found out at a social Christmas party, and it was Mrs. Gorgeous George herself who told me!

Evidently it was no secret that he was spending some of his money with me to get his extra gratification. His wife knew about it and entirely approved.

"So you're Xaviera?" she said when he introduced her to me at the party. "Please let me thank you for all the wonderful things you have done for my husband. You have improved our sex life enormously."

Mrs. Gorgeous George explained that after his sessions at my house, her husband was able to get aroused to the point that when he came home, he would lock her in a wrestling hold, put his penis in her, and ejaculate. Otherwise, she admitted to me, they never had any kind of sex.

I asked how he acquired his crazy hang-up, and she explained that when he was a scrawny twelve-year-old in school, a fat girl whom he had a kind of crush on picked him up in the gym one day, held him over her head for a minute, then dropped him to the floor, and laughed her insides out.

Her husband, she said, felt very humiliated, but at the same time he experienced a kind of sexual exhilaration, and when he reached manhood he started looking around for fat or hefty women.

She claimed, and it could be true, that he even hung around fairgrounds and circus sideshows having fantasies about the fat freak ladies. However, until he met me he never found anyone who combined attractive looks with strength and who would cooperate with him.

At the time I met his wife, I had already stopped seeing Gorgeous George, because I could not afford the time he took and did not enjoy walking around for the next two days after each session with stiff joints and a bruised body.

She implored me to start taking care of him again and even suggested I come to their big house, where there would be more space to wrestle. "If it would make you feel easier, I could always go out to my music lessons when you are there," she suggested.

I declined the offer.

Apart from the uncomfortable side effects, Gorgeous George's wrestling scene is a breeze compared to some of the unusual group scenes that have to be organized. To begin with, you often have to find and pay "extras" to participate, and that can sometimes border on disaster if you don't get the right one.

This happened in a group freak scene with a shy businessman named Lionel, who visited New York weekly.

Lionel was a voyeur who loved to watch movies of men making it together, or, better still, observe them at close quarters through a two-way mirror. He was a married man, but clearly he was a potential homosexual, and it would be only a matter of time before he plucked up the nerve to participate himself.

It happened one Sunday afternoon. "Xaviera, do you think it would be possible to arrange a nice, discreet young man for me to experiment with?" he asked sheepishly.

It was a very simple matter to phone up the stud service of Pim Anderson, who is also described as a madam, and ask him to send me over someone attractive and well hung.

And that's where you can get into difficulties using unknown studs.

With a girl you can see how she is built just by looking at her naked body, but if a stud says he has a big one, you have to take his word for it. You can't say, "Okay, let it all hang out."

This Sunday afternoon Pim sends me over a beautiful-looking kid named Raymond, who, just as the scene is about to begin, cannot get it up in the worst way.

I call him outside and ask him: "What's the problem, why can't you get it up?" And he says, "I already screwed five times today, and I also jerked off when I woke up this morning, because it felt so nice."

I can't use a tired stud, so I have to fire him. "If you want to be a stud on Sundays, don't jerk off, nut," I told him.

Meanwhile, poor Lionel has paid me $200, for which he

doesn't get a refund, but I promise him a fantastic four-way scene the next day. This time I get hold of Jonny Starr, the Negro from the umbrella store, who is in no way homosexual but whose cock is gigantic. Jonny will participate free of charge in almost anything as long as he gets the girl in the end.

Next afternoon, on my king-size bed are Lionel, Jonny, my roommate, Corinne, and me, and we're all waiting to go into the scene when Jonny stalls. Trouble again. His mammoth black cock lingers between the virgin white buttocks.

"I'm not going the Hershey Bar road without a rubber," he insists, and wants to delay the scene while I find one.

I can't find the damned rubber, so I say, "Listen, you're brown already, so what do you care?" And everybody laughs, and he agrees to go ahead anyway.

This time Lionel gets a really good scene. While he lies on his side, Corinne is in front of him giving him a blow job, and Jonny is behind him with his big cock going in and out while Lionel is screaming ow, ow, ow, ow, ow, because the first time it always hurts a lot. All the time I am behind Jonny, fingering his asshole and thinking a hard man is good to find.

In the end, Lionel is sore but ecstatic, Jonny has screwed both me and Corinne free of charge, and everybody has got their money's worth. However, two days later Lionel calls up to tell me that his square country wife is demanding to know why he has to eat his dinner off the mantelpiece.

If someone has a hang-up for weird group scenes, he will some-times go to all lengths to pursue them, and can even end up in a very dangerous situation, which is what happened to Nijinski, the guy who digs watching naked girls do ballet.

When I first met Nijinski I was a loner about to go into the madam business, and he wanted only one girl at a time. She had to cavort around in front of the mirror before they made love.

By a coincidence, I found out he lived in the same building where I opened my first house, and he became a regular customer, getting gradually kinkier. He used to put me through hoops finding non-Caucasian girls: Orientals, Negroes, anything but straight-up Anglo-Saxon types. Then he started insisting I give him a reduction in the fee because he was a regular customer.

In a way, I liked him; he was a brilliant graphic designer who worked with a leading advertising agency, but he would sometimes get on my nerves with his demands.

One Friday night around 4:00 A.M. when I had just gone to bed there was a persistent ringing of the doorbell. I went out and opened it to find Nijinski in the company of two vicious-looking black street whores, and he begged me to ask them in. "Hey, I want you to get to know my two new girlfriends," he said drunkenly. "They're very good ballet dancers."

"If they're ballet dancers, I'm an astronaut," I told him. "Good night, I am going back to sleep."

That night I had sent one of my girls, Elaine, out on a date for the whole night, and expected her back at eight the next morning with the check. I am the one who is always responsible for the check, and I pay the girl whether it bounces or not, but in this case I did not anticipate any difficulty because the client was the respected dean of a big university.

At eight the doorbell rang, and I opened it to find a trembling, semihysterical Elaine standing there white as a sheet.

"There are police and photographers all over the lobby," she said. "And the elevator is covered in blood."

I told her to calm down and gave her a cup of coffee, put on sunglasses and a wig, and went downstairs to investigate the matter. From the doorman I learned it was Nijinski, who was in critical condition in Bellevue Hospital.

On the way back to my apartment, I noticed blood smeared all over the hallway walls.

Some days later, when he was off the critical list, I decided to visit my friend in the hospital to see how he was and what had happened. He told me that when they got home, he'd asked the girls to disrobe and do some ballet steps for him. But they refused and demanded quick money instead.

"C'mon, we don't need that bullshit," they said "Give us a quick screw and a hundred dollars."

Nijinski, being drunk, offered to give them a check because he didn't have enough money. Now, the rules of the business are that street whores never accept checks, so when he started slowly writing it out, they got mad, grabbed a bread knife from the kitchen, and lunged at him.

Together they held him down, stuffed a handkerchief in his mouth, and blindfolded him. They broke a Coke bottle and buried the jagged end in his face, smashed the legs off the coffee table and used them to brutally beat him. Then they kicked his body and his balls and finally stabbed him repeatedly with the bread knife, and today he still has the ugly scars under his heart, on his abdomen, and around his throat.

The girls fled when he passed out, but not before taking with them everything of value they could carry from the apartment.

Mercifully he regained consciousness and managed to drag himself along the hall, and the last thing he remembered was pressing the elevator button with his chin before tumbling into the opening door.

Nijinski is a very subdued man now and leads a secluded life, but that terrible experience has not cured him of his hang-up. However, he is very careful whom he conducts his erotic ballet sessions with these days and has definitely changed his taste in "professional" ballerinas.

There is one other category of client with whom I definitely would prefer never having to do business: the ones whose hang-up is filth.

Their scenes include anything from messy meals to urine to feces, to put it bluntly, and even though they are willing to pay a fortune for their scene, I usually turn them down unless they can conduct their repulsive activities someplace other than my house.

One famous televison producer wants to pay through the nose for what girls do through the bladder—the golden shower.

This man was quite straight when I first met him, and I saw him gradually go from wanting the vibrator on his penis to the dildo in his anus, and finally one day asking me to urinate on him.

In time this became obsessive, and one day he called me and said, "Xaviera, I've been dreaming about having a dozen pretty girls pee all over me, and I will pay anything you ask if you would arrange it."

In those days I was not a madam yet, and I had lots of trouble rounding up eight girls who would participate. Then my boyfriend, Larry, had to go buy some plastic and rubber sheets to protect my bed, because the scene was to be held at my place.

The girls had been warned, before they came over, not to go to the bathroom, and were promised a $25 bonus on top of the $50 fee for the one who peed the longest. Just for good measure, I told them to drink a lot of beer before leaving for my place.

The producer arrived slightly crocked and drank half a bottle of Scotch before he lay naked on the waterproofed bed, and the bizarre scene began. All this time the movie projector was showing blue films on the wall, and now I sat on a chair with the stopwatch to time the girls as the first one came in and stood astride him and relieved herself.

Then the second, third, and fourth girls performed. Urine was starting to overflow on my bed and onto the floor, and I was getting fed up with the nauseating spectacle.

By the time the last girl had gone, the place looked like a pigsty, with puddles around the floor and pee in the producer's hair, eyes—everywhere. A little Puerto Rican girl with a bladder infection won the contest by maintaining a weak dribble for sixty-five seconds.

But he still hadn't had a climax, so I took the biggest dildo around and jammed it in his rear end, and he popped his cookies. Then I threw him in the tub with lots of Badedas and scrubbed him all over, took him out, and dried him off, then remembered I had not washed his hair, and had to bathe him all over again.

The beer, the birds, and the bath cost him $800, and he was pleased to pay the price. However, I didn't want my house turned into a public urinal ever again, so I sent him to a rival madam.

Mr. Filthy Rich is something else again. This incredibly handsome, intelligent, charming, and wealthy man wants you to feed him your shit—literally—with a silver spoon out of a plate. One girl I know makes a fortune by telephoning him when she feels the urge, and he always tells her to get in a cab and come right over.

But most of my girls don't like going there, easy money though it is, because at thirty-two, Mr. Filthy Rich is so handsome and would make some girl such a gorgeous lover that they can't bring themselves to do what he wants.

One more thing that especially bothers me about Mr. Filthy Rich is that the crockery he uses for his revolting deviation is a blue Delft plate—my country's most treasured export!

Henry the Eighth is one of the heaviest filth freaks in the whole of my black book and has been thrown out of every respectable hotel in New York because he is such a big pig.

In truth, he looks more like a frog than a pig. He's a repulsive man with olive eyes that sort of pop out of his head, and a fat, slobbery mouth.

If a girl is smart, she can get a lot of money from him, but it takes a lot of patience and a strong stomach. This big, fat slob's hang-up is ordering huge quantities of food up to his room and wolfing it down while he gets stoned on grass, cocaine, amyl nitrate, and other stimulants.

He pushes it all into his mouth in large fistfuls while grunting and snorting like a pig; then, when he can't fit any more into his mouth, he starts hurling it around the room. He throws peas, carrots, chicken bones, gravy, all over the room, in the light fixtures, the draperies, the girl even catches it on her dress, and, of course, there's food all over the bed.

Then, depending on how freaky his mood is, he wants the girl to kick him, slap him, tie him down, spit in his face, and sometimes even pee on him. Finally he gets his rocks off when the girl uses a strong vibrator on his penis while he is slobbering with his liver-lips on her vagina.

You can imagine the screams the maids let out when they come in to clean up his room next morning.

It's a repulsive scene, but of course he means well; he's just a big baby. However, that's not the way the hotel managers look at his behavior, and that is why he has eaten his way through every hotel in Manhattan.

When Henry the Eighth first called me up, he had a suite in the Plaza. Last time I heard from him was from a rundown motel on Tenth Avenue in the Twenties.

One famous movie director was the master of the macabre both on and off the screen. He had a room in his California villa specially equipped as a funeral parlor, and he would lie in an open coffin of polished mahogany with heavy brass handles, surrounded by banks of flowers. He was made up in a deathly pallor and wore a silk shroud. His secretary would be sent to find a couple of girls, preferably not professionals, and they would be led into the darkened room, where tall candles burned at the foot of the bier. The place was filled with soft organ music, and the girls would peer inside the coffin to pay their last respects. The "corpse" lay with his hands folded, not over his stomach but clutching his penis. As they leaned over, he would raise his body and open his eyes. At the moment that the girls ran screaming from the room, they would each be handed an envelope containing a hundred dollars, and he would reach his orgasm.

Fourteen

The Business of Pleasure

*E*veryone seems to think that high-class prostitutes, especially madams, have a lot of money. Lawyers in particular must believe this, because they always charge me three or four times what they would charge a regular client for their time and effort.

Now it is true that my business—as my stockbroker would put it—*does* generate a large cash flow. The top madams in town can make $5,000 a week during a good week in January, February, and March, but the rest of the year it's much more likely to be $3,000 a week. And expenses are large year-round.

I almost always have five or six girls working in my three-bedroom apartment from Monday night through Thursday night. On weekends, however, the johns desert New York and go back to their families in Long Island, Ohio, or wherever they are from. Summer weekends, they take off as early as Thursday to go out to the Hamptons.

In addition to the girls at the apartment, I am usually sending another five girls out to apartments and hotel rooms each night. Some customers, and this is particularly true of Latins, want to make a big occasion out of seeing one of my girls. Dinner, champagne, a floor show—these johns want to lavish on the prostitute before fucking her. So I won't send a girl out on a three-hour dinner date for under two hundred dollars. But the rich South Americans have their own style and don't mind paying to maintain it.

Most of my customers come to me as a result of word-of-mouth publicity. If somebody arrives at my place and he looks like a wealthy man and can spend large sums of money, I'll first of all ease the price up above my fifty-dollar minimum. If I think he can go for more money, I give him two or three girls and, bending my rule, let him pay up front. For a trip-around-the-world, if indeed the girl is willing to perform this intimate service with her tongue around the john's behind, we usually charge double. If he hasn't enough cash with him, I accept a check, even if he's new to my place. You can tell if a man is wealthy.

When a man leaves my place, and he's from a city like Washington, Chicago, or Philadelphia, and not New York, I give him a few of my interior-decorator cards and ask him to give them out to his business friends and tell them to just call me any time.

When a Texan walks into my place, the price is immediately a C-note—a hundred dollars. They generally are the best-spending customers I get. For his money a customer is entitled to half an hour with a girl—and no money back if not delighted.

We squeeze in the stockbrokers for a quick fifty dollars. They're not demanding because they're always horny. They come up often, and they're not the type to hang around for three hours drinking up my booze. Basically they're very easygoing and fast.

Sometimes I get men who are impotent and want to eat up two or three girls while still not being able to come. They waste a lot of time and are usually the ones who give me a hard time when it's time to pay. But most of my customers get their rocks off in much less time than the allotted half an hour. Then if they want another go, even with the same girl, and even within the thirty minutes they must pay again.

Lately I split fifty-fifty with my girls, and every night is pay day. The girls I send over to hotel rooms usually come back to me each night after they've finished work to give me my 50 percent madam's fee. Sometimes, however, they are so tired that it is not until the next day they bring my money to me. Almost always, my outside girls are honest and split fairly with me. Since both they and their customers need me, they generally don't cheat. For instance, if I send a girl to a hotel room and instead of only one fuck, she makes the customer climax three times, she could collect $150, and tell me he came only once. But this almost never happens, especially since the customer likes to remind me how much he's paying me. Maybe he hopes I will give him a discount someday.

A lot of men seem to wake up horny in the morning and would like to see me but can't get to my place. For them I have a special service. I let them telephone me, and I talk them into an orgasm while they jerk off. For this I usually don't get paid, but I know they'll be back as paying customers some night.

But to tell the truth, I am trying to stop this service now, because I am usually up until five in the morning carrying out the administrative duties of a madam, and just getting my beauty sleep when these horny guys wake me up.

Some of the girls live in my apartment for a week or month at a time. For this they pay me $125 a week, and, of course, they get the first choice of the clients who come in—especially the nooners, who want a quick fuck or a blow job at lunchtime. So the girls don't object to this rent arrangement, and it helps me, because large apartments always run $500 to $1,000 a month.

In order to keep my business lively and growing, I have had to adopt that very American system of credit. For instance, one of the biggest stockbrokerage houses on Wall Street has a credit rating with me of up to two thousand dollars. They send their best out-of-town executives and customers up to me, and once a week the vice president puts the cash owed me in an envelope and sends it to me with a messenger from the firm.

I take a lot of my payments in personal checks, but this, of course, can be risky. As in any other business, it is impossible to completely escape bad checks and bad accounts.

I keep a little red book in which I record my operating accounts. On the left side of the page I list the customers by name and how much they pay. On the right side of the page are the names of the girl or girls each john saw. This way I can be sure each girl gets paid correctly. I also know how much came in each day. In the back of the book I keep a list of my charge customers and how much they owe me. I also keep a list of the checks that bounce, so I can have Larry, my boyfriend, try to collect for me.

Also in the red book I keep a record of the money I invest. On Christmas and birthdays, I send my parents lovely presents. Until my name was splashed in newspapers all over the world after I got involved in a New York corruption scandal, my mother fondly believed that I was still working for the Dutch consulate. Then one day she found herself gazing at a picture of her dear daughter, brandishing a whip and looking as if she were intent on scaring the life out of the photographer. She blamed herself for somehow failing me, and it was many years before I could convince her that I had not become a hooker in order to avenge myself on my parents. My father had become very ill and, fortunately, did not realize what had been going on. As I was constantly being chased from one apartment to another by the police, I had taken the precaution of having all my mail addressed to Larry's office.

Whenever I find I have more than a thousand dollars in cash lying around, I telephone Larry and say, "I just saw George" or "George was here." That means I have a G, a thousand dollars, to go into the box. I have to be careful on the phones, because frequently I find they are tapped.

But now, let me show you the other side of the ledger. My huge outlay.

In the back of my red book I see that I am owed $8,000 in credit accounts and checks that have bounced. I will be lucky if I collect $3,500 of that money. My yearly loss because of maltreatment in business is more than 20 percent of my total earnings.

If my business was legitimate, I could write off some of the crippling costs of my lifestyle as expenses. And my hectic life affects me physically as well as financially. When I look in the mirror, I see how tired I am. But I have great reserves of energy and a zest for life which enables me to shake off any bitterness and I refuse to let myself become miserable. I don't drink or smoke, and I take frequent trips to such places as Las Vegas or Puerto Rico, where I acquire a great suntan and keep my good looks along with my good health.

I trust Larry absolutely, and he stashes away my cash in various safe deposits, to which I hold duplicate keys.

So, as I say, to begin with I have a 20 percent loss off the top, and that represents a 10 percent cash outlay, because every night I pay my girls in cash their half of what they earn, even if I accept a check or let the customer charge.

My biggest outlay is when the police raid my apartment and arrest me and my girls. So far this year I have had three disastrous busts. One was in March, a second in April, and a third in late July. Each time I am busted I have to bail out myself and all my girls, pay the fines against us, and, most of all, pay the lawyers. This is not counting what I pay off to the police. These payoffs averaged over $1000 per month and were spread all over the precinct. Once or twice police officers told me they quashed complaints, but the fact is I have just been forced to move for the fourth time in less than a year.

After every bust, I have to move to a new apartment in a different precinct. That means moving vans, new wall-to-wall carpeting, having the phones reinstalled, and trying to get the business going again at a new address.

So now maybe you get a better idea of some of the expenses big madams are faced with. Just the ordinary expenses of running a house like mine are high. I have a maid every night, sometimes a butler, and the liquor my customers drink also runs up.

In my business we also have unusual petty-cash expenditures, which can become large items. Take for instance the large-size lingerie, black fishnet tights, panties, bras, garter belts, leather goods, and wigs I have to buy and keep in my closet for the transvestites who want to be all dressed up by me and the girls. These delicate feminine underthings don't last long, being stretched out of shape by the men who wear them. And the frilly things have to be washed constantly, because these clients usually come all over them or in them. But lawyers and payoffs are what hit me the hardest. In the last eight months they have come to about $25,000.

I paid $400 to the police just to get back my black book after my last arrest. This book, which I have brought up to date myself, is the heart of my business. Just as I keep all my financial records in my red book, in the black book I keep all the information about my customers: names, addresses, telephone numbers. If I have a home phone number, I put it in brackets to remind me not to call unless in an emergency like a bounced check. I keep little notes on the johns, such as whether they spend $50 or $100, if they want two girls at a time, drink a lot, weirdo, slave, con artist, big cock, sweet person, shy, likes variety, likes to eat pussy, pays extra for around-the-world, and COD—that means get paid up front, he's stingy or tries to chisel you down.

A typical entry in my book would look like this: "Peter Pan; . . ; OK; Lolitas; diminutive."

Translated, this means that the john called Peter Pan pays ' . . '—which is code for $50. His credit is good (OK). He likes very young girls (Lolitas). He has a small cock (diminutive). Another john in my book is coded as follows: "Steve Super-cock;*; COD; Groups; SF."

Steve's name in the book speaks for itself as to the size of his cock. He pays '*'—or $100. His credit isn't too good, and he haggles about price, so get the money up front (COD). He likes making the scene with more than one girl at a time (Groups). He's an out-of-towner from San Francisco (SF).

If I put down "M/S" after a name, the guy is a slave, and I get out my goodie bag when he comes over. Sometimes I have the real name of a customer in the book followed by his pseudonym.

But in any case I know who all of them really are, but go along with their desire to be called by the fake name they have taken. So it is easy to see why I can't afford to lose my books, which are really the most valuable things I own. I have to get them back, and naturally I pay off if I have to.

Another important service also costs me much more than it should. In my four moves this past year, I went through the same real-estate agent. This guy is socking it to me on fees and commissions, he cheats me left and right, but I stay with him because he always gives me a cool building. He knows the manager of the building, he knows the superintendent, and he knows that there are other girls working in the building. All this is so important to me that I cannot argue about being hit over the head with expenses. And my real-estate broker will take nothing out in trade with me.

I use this expression, "take it out in trade," a lot. I do indeed operate on a barter basis. A man who runs a private country club in New Jersey brings me most of my liquor in cases that he takes out of the club's liquor supply. I give him a girl for a case of liquor and pay the girl $25. This man is usually quite horny, and once he wanted five girls in a night. He gave me three cases of liquor and a check for $100. My florist gave me two big, beautiful indoor plants worth $80 for one quickie. My jeweler gives me a good discount for a screw now and again, and there is even this old Jewish shoemaker down on Ninth Street who makes the finest shoes and takes his pay in a girl. He made me a beautiful pair easily worth $50, and when I came to get them he put me in the chair of his dirty little office. I only took my pants off, put my legs up and apart, and the old cobbler got it up enough to get in me. Wham-bam, thank you, ma'am! In less than two minutes, he came and I went off with the shoes.

A furniture manufacturer I know gave me two chairs and a chaise longue for a few blow jobs, and even the staff of the Chinese restaurant downstairs in my building brings up Chinese food at a discount. In return I give these Chinese boys a girl for half-price, $25. This is in addition to their once-a-month freebie in exchange for free meals.

I tip the five doormen in the building $20 a week, but the superintendent prefers that I give him a girl twice a month, which in my system of accounting is worth $100. The building manager I tip on the same basis, so it costs me $200 a month in trade to take care of the two of them. These gifts are worthwhile, because after an arrest a prostitute gets evicted right away, but this didn't happen to me after my last, well-publicized arrest. I screwed the manager an extra time and as a special favor fucked one of his friends as well. Thus I was allowed to stay in my apartment until I was ready to move at leisure into a new place.

It is always important to be friendly with the building personnel. I remember I came home from a friend's party one night very horny, and this tall seventeen-year-old Negro boy was on duty at the entrance to the building. I told him to come up to my apartment so I could give him his tip. He came up, and I almost raped him. We fucked our brains out, plus I gave him $10, and so he was quite happy with his tip. Trouble was, he fell in love with me. For me it was no more than washing my hands. Once I had him, I forgot him, but he kept calling me and giving me presents, such as records and flowers, and I had a hard time discouraging him from bothering me.

I also have a swinging druggist who gives me amyl nitrate without prescription and lets me have a good rate on the KY jelly and cosmetics I buy in quantity. Although I have never fucked the druggist, he sometimes sends me his special friends, whom I take care of. One of my girlfriends has a beautifully furnished apartment, and she literally fucked it together. Everything in the apartment she got by screwing manufacturers and salesmen.

As I mentioned, one of my main expenses is having my four telephones installed each time I have to move to a new apartment. This is a big job and takes two or three days, since I have a set of wall phones plus others in two locations. Fortunately, I have a friend at the telephone company: a telephone installer I call when I need him. He comes over himself and does the job, and I pay him handsomely—or fuck him myself when he finishes.

While I was working for Madeleine, I discovered a girl can even trade her way around the world. I mean traveling in an airplane. Madeleine came from South Africa, and she liked to go back to visit, except the trip was expensive: about $1,200 first class. One of her best customers was a very horny guy who was one of the owners of a major airline. For her round-trip ticket she would give this guy girls worth the amount of the ticket, and thus, even after paying the girls their share, she saved 50 percent on the price of the trip.

When I started my own business, this same guy came to me and wanted to trade tickets for my girls. I said I would work something out with him when I was ready to go to Holland again, but at the moment, I preferred cash payments. This sort of trade deal is really worthwhile if you want to take a long trip to Hawaii or Australia. Then you can really feel the difference in working out the tickets in trade.

One travel agent who did indeed send me customers used to come around and want a girl for free. I have never been tempted to give it away free to someone just because he sends me customers. Once you start that, everybody wants a freebie for bringing in new customers. Then it starts to snowball, and soon you're screwing everybody for free. The travel agent tried to be businesslike. He pointed out that for every ten tickets he sold to Europe he got one for himself free. I told him I was very sorry, but I could not compete with the airline's incentive program.

Nevertheless, at Christmastime, when some of my really big spenders call me, I may give them a freebie myself as a sort of present. And last Christmas I thought it was appropriate to send out a tasteful Christmas card to my customers and at the same time remind them of my existence and give them my latest address. After Christmas I received quite a few phone calls from men who thanked me for letting them know my new number and where I was.

So this, then, is the story of my income and outlay as New York's biggest madam. I think it proves that if my business could be made legal, the way off-track betting is in New York, I and women like me could make a big contribution to what Mayor John Lindsay calls Fun City, and the city and state could derive the money in taxes and licensing fees that I pay off to crooked cops and political figures. Since the beginning of time, no government has ever stopped prostitution, because men want it. The proof of this is that my best clients represent the highest echelon of government and business circles and keep me in business no matter how often I am harassed by the police and have to change addresses.

I have always carried on my business openly as if it were legal. However, after several brushes with the law, I had to become more circumspect. They called me the European Madam, since prostitution is more tolerated in most European countries than in the States. Of course, American official condemnation is phony. Hypocrites in public life denounce immorality, yet leaders of the business, entertainment, and political communities were among my best clients. Even though I have been thrown in jail a number of times, I have refused to disclose the true names of my clients. The tax authorities went through my telephone accounts with a fine-tooth comb and went so far as to pursue me to Holland to demand the identity of who it was I used to call at the White House. Since I had quit the States, I was able to refuse to divulge that mouth-watering item of scandal.

In my opinion, it is ridiculous that prostitution should be treated as a crime. How can it be a crime when there is no victim? There are abuses, but so are there in other professions, and it is legal harassment which encourages those sordid hookers whose pimps beat up their clients. You don't find that sort of thing in the relaxed atmosphere of a well-run brothel or in the activities of private call girls. Why should not girls who take proper pains over hygiene and who are honest with their clients be permitted to work legally, like any other social worker?

After I had ceased to be the Happy Hooker and was living in Canada, I acted as a consultant with the Clarks Institute of Sexology in Toronto. It was not that I acted as a surrogate lover—I hardly ever slept with anyone I met doing this work—but very often specially difficult cases which were referred to me would speak openly, whereas they would clam up with the doctors or psychiatrists. There were youths who were convicted rapists and child molesters who admitted to me that if they had enjoyed access to sexual partners, some of their crimes would never have been committed.

Fifteen

For Pleasure
More Than Profit

The old saying "Never mix business with pleasure" does not always apply to the business of pleasure.

If I didn't have my heart literally in my work, or sometimes fall in love, I would go crazy. For example, I was in Miami that lonely Christmas after Carl left me, as the houseguest of a swinging New York socialite, Dennis Tanner, and his bitchy Swedish wife. After she fell asleep at night, he would come to my room and make love to me till dawn. However, I wanted somebody for myself, to share the holiday fun with, a man to escort me around the parties and private clubs.

One evening a group of us went to a place called the Palm Bay Club, which was rather stuffy but quite good fun. Even though my hosts made a point of including me in the conversation and the dancing, I was feeling acutely lonely. Once in a while I would do a little reconnaissance trip around the room, but the attractive men were all attached.

Toward the end of the evening, as I stood near the bar alone, my famous orange juice in my hand, the reveling crowd around me parted like the Sea of Galilee and out walked one of the most gorgeous men I had seen in Miami—alone.

He was so stunningly glamorous, he looked like the classic *Cosmopolitan* fiction illustration of the lover. His immaculate white suit accentuated his even suntan, and his face was crowned with black hair cut in Roman-boy style and rakishly long. I guessed him to be in his late thirties. He had, I hoped, a stranger's lost look in his eyes.

As the man walked closer to me, our eyes embraced, and something compelled us to touch each other's arm. I spoke first. "Are you as lonely as I am?" I asked.

"I guess I am," he replied, to my utter joy, "and I could use some charming feminine company." With zero resistance from me, he took my arm and steered me from the Palm Bay Club, into a taxi, and on to a more swinging discothèque called the Penthouse, where we laughed and danced and talked German together until around three in the morning.

His name was Paul Lindfeld, and he was a famous New York jewelery designer of German-Jewish extraction, recently divorced. When the evening wound up, he took me to the Jockey Club, where he was staying, and without too many words we slipped into his bed and made love.

We turned on to each other's bodies so intensely and became so passionate that the people in the next room started complaining and knocking on the wall. But we just ignored them and continued our lovemaking.

Before we fell asleep exhausted I knew this was a man I could really seriously fall in love with, and before the relationship went any further I would have to tell him the truth about who I was and what I did.

I didn't think he would take the news too badly, since he was a sophisticated kind of man. I felt he could accept my professional status for what it was.

"Paul, there is something I think you ought to know about me," I said.

"I know already," he said sleepily. "You're wonderful in bed."

"Thank you for the compliment," I said, "but the matter is slightly more serious than that. You see, if I weren't good in bed I would be out of business, if you know what I mean."

"What exactly do you mean?" he asked, wide-awake now.

"I am trying to tell you that I am not exactly what you believe I am—the little interior designer on her annual vacation. I am actually a professional woman—a call girl."

He sat bolt upright and backed off.

Before he could speak, I continued, "Please don't think I am going to ask you to pay me, or anything like that. I wasn't working tonight. With you it was true desire."

Paul was visibly jolted by the revelation but we talked about it a little more, and he accepted it unconditionally.

The next morning I moved out of the Tanners' house and in with Paul. We spent every moment of the next few days together inseparable as Siamese twins. It was the first time I had felt like this in ages, despite all my experiences. Forget about Evelyn St. John—this was much deeper. We went everywhere together, and he was so handsome and charming that I wore him on my sleeve like a *croix de guerre*.

Back in New York, after a long, depressing period of not hearing from Paul, I finally did get a call from him explaining how busy he'd been, and we took over from where we left off in Miami. Paul lived on the twenty-fifth floor of an apartment building on Central Park South, and the winter panorama outside across the snow-covered park was pure Grandma Moses and terribly romantic. The apartment was elegant, expensive, and tastefully decorated with antiques. The bedroom had an oval-shaped window and the view blew my mind.

Paul was in wonderful condition, his cock was precious but not too big, and he was basically a square lover. But we didn't need gimmicks of any kind. Variations are there usually if you're getting slightly bored with the normal position. However, when it's love, the normal position is as exciting as standing on your head and doing it.

The feelings I had at that moment for Paul were almost as deep as those I had had for Carl. I guess this was the first time since Carl I had felt this way, because I had been hurt so badly that I didn't want to give myself any more pain. In a way, I had grown up, matured. And maturity comes with suffering and experience in life, I believe.

I had a second telephone installed in my apartment exclusively for his calls, and his ego was flattered by that. I was working as a single then, so I could easily take nights off. Sometimes we would go to the theater and dinner, and always we would return to his apartment.

About a month after we started our blazing affair, Paul wanted me to let him make love to me Greek style. I had never done that before, and I resisted.

But Paul was persistent. "You've done everything in your life. You've been a prostitute, and before that you've had a lot of men, so if you love me, let me take your virginity in the only remaining place."

I loved him, so I let him do it his way.

Paul was strangely excited by the acquisition of my ass, and he got very carried away. He had a rhythm that really shakes your bowels, and he made me unbelievably sore. From that night on he would regularly want me to let him do it that way. In the beginning it kept hurting, but after a while I even started enjoying it now and then, since luckily he wasn't too big for me.

Still and all, he gave no thought to my pleasure. *His* desires were the ones that had to come first, whether I liked it or not. I started recognizing in Paul traits that were disturbingly reminiscent of Carl. Along with his selfish sexuality, Paul was not at all generous—even stingier than Carl had been in New York. Even on a cold winter night, he wouldn't part with cab fare. This turned me off in a way, even though I still cared for him deeply. I slowly began to see other things in my Adonis too. Even though he wanted the comfort of a steady girlfriend, he wanted the freedom as well, and he was not really the type of man to be tied down by one woman. Since the road to love started becoming slightly rocky, I found myself with free time on my hands and started circulating among a crowd of swinging friends to distract me from my disappointment in our affair.

One evening I made a date to meet a group of friends at a bar on First Avenue called My House. My House has a front piano bar and a back room where I was to join the crowd.

As I picked my way through the place, I caught sight of a girl with blond hair and a round face who looked strangely like me. The trace of narcissism that exists in all of us attracted me to her.

As I got very close, I heard her speak in a sultry voice, and I knew I would love to make it with her. Although she didn't look like a swinger, the man with her did, so my strategy was to approach him first.

I went around behind him and whispered in his ear. "Hi, my name is Xaviera, and I am going to make a suggestion that I hope won't offend you," I said. "I would really love to be with you and your girl in a swing—preferably just your girl. Is there any possibility?"

I could see he loved the idea. He smiled mysteriously, then whispered to his girlfriend, and she reacted with shock and retreated into her shell and said nothing.

"Look, if my suggestion will cause any jealousy or ill feeling, just tell me, and I'll take off. But if you would like to join me and come to a party being given by a close friend, an important politician from Albany, you can think it over." I said. I saw the eagerness in his eyes.

"If you like the idea, we'll take it from there. If you don't, then you can leave from the party," I continued.

At the horny boyfriend's urging they both joined me. His name was Marvin, hers was Lisa, and they had been dating each other for about two years, although both were married to different partners.

We stayed at the party a couple of hours, during which I took every opportunity to turn Lisa on. And the way you can turn a woman on, or at least tell if she is a sexual type, is to stroke the inside of her arms, or in her hair, or on the back of her neck. If you are sitting down at a table, you can reach down and stroke behind her legs. A sensual woman always reacts to this.

Mellowed by a few drinks at the party, and semiseduced by me, Lisa and Marvin decided to leave for my apartment around midnight.

Before we left, I also picked up a big, square Texan who looked very bored and very rich. "If you pay me one hundred dollars," I told the Texan, "you'll have a better time than you're

having here. In fact, you might even have one of the most exciting nights of your life. I can promise you a fantastic swing," I
went on, "and you can watch me make it with this girl or you can
participate, and you may even fuck me or her."

I don't usually take somebody from a party and try to turn
him into a john, but in this case I recognized the possibility of
combining business with pleasure.

Marvin and Lisa I would never charge, of course, because I
liked them as friends. They were for pleasure more than profit.

By the time we reached my apartment, Lisa had dropped her
inhibitions and started slowly undressing, until she was completely nude. Her body was voluptuous, not unlike a Rubens
painting, soft and full. Her breasts were not all that big, but they
were firm and erect, her lips were moist and tender, her tongue
was hungry for sex. Her eyes had a faraway look, knowing what
she could expect to come and yet with a childlike innocence.

I brushed my eager lips against her mouth, her cheeks and
nose, while circling her shell-formed ears with my warm tongue.
She stiffened and sighed, goose bumps appearing on her arms
and legs. My hands reached up to massage the back of her head,
and then down to her neck, while her silky blond hair slipped
through my fingers like sand on a beach. We both stepped back,
and like falling on a cloud, we stretched ourselves out on my
bed.

A fierce desire for her inviting body made my blood course
through my body, and I reached with one hand to her left breast,
at the same time caressing her right nipple with my tongue. Lisa,
meanwhile, like a kitten beginning to wake for dinner, started to
moan softly. With one hand she nudged my head lower and
lower, until she rooted it to the source of her greatest pleasure.
With my fingers I gently opened the petals of her sweet flower,

and her body moved upward and outward to open a larger door to our pleasurable play. And once opened, there was no way back. My tongue darted in and out, exciting her more and more.

Marvin and the Texan, meanwhile, were watching in anticipation, all excited by the view of this loving scene. They both climbed on the queen-size bed, but it became too crowded, so I ordered them: "Get off, please, I want to be alone with my girl." And they did. All of a sudden I felt like a man trying to protect his girl.

I know exactly where to find the clitoris, better often than many a man. You open the top of the woman's vagina, and there, sometimes hidden away, you will find, like a miniature penis, the little clitoris. It contains the same number of nerves as the male equivalent, so it is intensely sensitive. It also gets a hard-on like a penis, and it is a matter of vibrating your tongue, finger, or vibrator, putting the passionate feeling into the little clitoris to make the woman climax. The little hard-on explodes, the clitoris disappears, and you can feel the whole body shake in ecstasy like a spastic movement, uncontrollable once it gets going.

As I concentrated on my new play toy, Lisa, her body seemed to me to give forth an aroma of honeysuckle in the spring, and the taste of her was like honey to this hungry bee. As I stimulated her clitoris, her hands sought my head to explore deeper and deeper. All of a sudden I felt the urge to be a man, if only I could fill the deeper void that lay within! In quickening strokes she lifted her body and encircled my head with her thighs, until her body poured out to me, and my cheeks and lips became moist.

Lisa and I awoke as if from a dream and became aware of our male companions. Almost immediately Marvin frantically went down on me while the Texan made love to Lisa. We were perspiring, and our bodies made squishy-squishy noises. Breathing was loud, mixed with moans from me and the delicate, passionate Lisa.

The combinations and appetites were inexhaustible, and it was almost morning before the bewildered Texan, not quite believing what had happened, dressed and left. After Marvin and Lisa departed, I slept, utterly fulfilled.

And that was the beginning of a swinging period for me, even though I was going steady with Paul and was still very much in love with him.

However, the syndrome was disconcertingly similar to the Carl affair. As with Carl, I confessed the episode with Lisa and Marvin to Paul, more or less hoping he would realize what he was driving me to. But instead of commiserating, his first words were: "When can we all get together?"

Paul had never been in a swing, and I should have made sure it stayed that way. I had had enough bitter experience to know that converting straights into swingers usually pushes them past the point of no return.

But in order to please Paul, I organized a dinner date with the couple, after which we all went back to his apartment. I had to orchestrate the scene, and even though my heart wasn't in an orgy, I did not want to be regarded as the wet blanket.

We pulled Paul's bed out into the middle of the room and all piled on naked and started caressing each other: I kissed Paul's nipples, intending gradually to work my way down to his penis, but when I got there, Lisa the shrinking violet had already arrived.

She was sucking him as if her life depended on it, and the two of them were so engrossed with each other that I was suddenly quite jealous at being excluded. I can swing happily enough with people with whom I am not emotionally involved, but when I really love a man I cannot bear to share him with some casual friend. So the sight of Paul sucking, fucking, and eating Lisa's delicious pussy upset me so much that I stalked out of the room, only to be followed by Marvin, who started to kiss me, but I was in no mood to appreciate his slobbery attentions. Finally I got so uptight that I invited everyone to depart and leave Paul alone with me. It was still early, and my insistence was not by any means popular with my guests, while Paul was in a surly mood for the rest of the night.

We only had a few precious nights left, but they were spoiled by Paul's continually asking me to invite in a girlfriend. Yet I loved the guy so much that I went out of my way to turn straight friends into swingers just to please him. The scene got so tense that, on one occasion, I had to explain to a girl that she was the one who had to leave my apartment, not me.

The strain of the gradual breakdown of our relationship together with professional worries was telling on me; I was becoming tense, irritable, and depressed. I saw less and less of Paul, but instead of my jealousy growing, my mental exhaustion and my disappointment at his selfishness turned me apathetic to the point at which I provided him with girls without feeling any pangs. All that was left were the amusing hours we would still spend chatting and joking on the phone. My physical desire for him had totally vanished, but at least I was able to enjoy him as a disembodied voice.

Sixteen

Ships in the Night

The last time I got busted, the New York newspapers described one of my unfortunate lovers, Takis, as "Madam Xaviera's pimp." While this may have made good copy, it was hardly the truth. The truth is, modern madams of any stature don't have pimps.

Street hookers have pimps who live off girls' earnings. I don't deny there may be some fringe benefits attached to being the successful madam's boyfriend, but as a rule her earnings, as with any other businesswoman, are her own. Apart from gifts for specific occasions, I have never spent money on a man, and I prefer it the other way around. But in Madeleine's case, the man she made her fourth husband had an ex-wife and several kids to support, and she was very rich in real-estate investments and savings. My feeling there was that the poor little guy deserved some compensation for leaving his wife and kids.

Pimps are usually involved in gambling, drugs, and white slavery, and the pimp never wants the girl to get out of the business—unless she is no good at her work anymore.

The pimp is traditionally a polygamous animal who keeps several girls—"wives-in-law." The structure is somewhat family-like, with the pimp as the master and the girls in friendly competition. Girls with pimps are known to work harder and longer (sometimes around the clock), and the pimp collects all the money—and no cheating around, or else he beats them up. It seems to me that it must be some kind of animal instinct that makes these girls enslave themselves to one man this way. Yet some girls do try to hold out money, and if he suspects this is going on, he will make spot checks of his stable. The pimp supplies the necessities for his girls—rent, furniture, and clothing, this latter often purchased "hot" from others in the life. On weekends he often takes them out to show off—to various nightclubs and discothèques and the more famous after-hours places.

The madam's boyfriend, on the other hand, is generally monogamous. There is a rule in my house that the girls must respect the boyfriend, or lovers, of the madam, and any fooling around with "the old man" will result in instant dismissal of the girl.

In Georgette's case the situation is a weird reverse. Georgette's stockbroker boyfriend, Stephen, is interested only in drugs, booze, and broads, in that order. Her solution is to pay her own girls to sleep with him. That way, she rationalizes, he doesn't have to stray—at least not outside her front door. He is not really what you call a pimp, yet Georgette is always crying poverty. As stingy as she is to her girls, that's how generous she is to him. I'd estimate that 90 percent of her money goes to him—his "trips" and his girls.

In my house, the only one who cheats is me. My private life is like a perpetual triangle, with myself and my steady boyfriend, Larry, as the constant side, and the lovers who pass through— some quicker than others—as the variable third.

As I've said before, I am an emotional person. I have my ups and downs, and if my boyfriend weren't there, safe and sure, and if I didn't occasionally fall in love, I would get very depressed and couldn't keep my head straight.

In those days in New York, it was Larry who was always there, reliable and solid. He looked after my administrative problems, checked out guys who tried to move in on me, and was always a good lover. He would help around the house and not try to drag me out to football games or cocktail parties when what I needed was simply to relax at home after hours of exhausting work. Being a madam is no career for the lazy—not if you want to suc- ceed! So he was easy to have about and I trusted him absolutely, certainly more than I should have.

But even then, I realized that Larry was not the man with whom I could contentedly spend the rest of my days. I needed more intellectual stimulation, somebody who shared my interest in literature, the theater, and music, and a man who could be decisive and dominant, who would occasionally bang his fist on the table and lay down the law—a man whom I could not only love and adore but also respect.

But Larry has been an absolute darling, considering all that I put him through.

I have insulted him, hurt his feelings, and stepped on his heart. From time to time I have told Larry I am in love with someone, and many times I have cheated right under his nose. But I told him they are all just ships passing in the night.

I let him know about the time I dragged the Negro doorman

upstairs, screwed his pants off, and gave him a $10 tip because he really deserved it. And the time the dentist's laughing gas got me so horny I made him send the nurse on an errand, and we made love in the chair.

Larry got hurt and angry when I told him about these things, even though I have never led him to believe I am anything but promiscuous. I also tried to include him in some of the extra activity, but it was usually a failure because he got so jealous.

One time I took him to the nudist colony in New Jersey to join in the swinging there, and unfortunately for Larry, soon after we walked in I saw the beautifully shaped, suntanned behind of an attractive man, and there was nothing I would rather do than stick my tongue in between his buttocks. No pussy time today. My mood is man.

The man was a gym teacher named Phil who was at the camp with his not-too-attractive girlfriend, and they were both swingers looking for partners.

No problem, we were ready. At least I was. Larry was not turned on at all by the girl, and once inside their cabin he became petulant and just sat back there on the bed while she was going down on him. But not me: I was like a wolf after Phil's ass.

He had a fine; athletic body and surely knew how to use it. When I squatted beside him, he wrapped his legs firmly around my neck, and that put me in the perfect position to devour his delicious buttocks, and in no time he was returning the compliment. The more sensually my hips undulated, the more jealously Larry glared at me. But I was so ecstatic as I tantalized that superb cock and as my hard, erect clitoris responded to his vibrating tongue, that I was oblivious to Larry's displeasure and mounting anger.

For me, this is the most delicious way of making love to a man, if it is someone who knows what he is doing. But meanwhile, I have to eat his cock, feel that penis to such an extent that it is about to explode in my mouth. It is just as much a psychological as well as physical mixture. If a man lies between my legs and eats me, even though he may have a better angle of doing it, it does not turn me on as much as the mutual "lingus." It has to be a two-way street, and both parties should be enjoying each other equally.

With Phil, who had multiple orgasms, it was the most fantastic experience. I climaxed almost immediately, breaking a promise Larry and I had made, that in swings we could give our bodies, but not our orgasms. Larry just sat there grinding his teeth to a powder and making fists of his hands. His poor partner must have got an inferiority complex when his usually big hard-on melted like an ice-cream pop.

Luckily Larry shut up until Phil and I had reached our climax, and then the fireworks started. "You did not keep your promise not to climax with another man. You even ate his ass, and you never eat mine!" he raged.

I suppose that last accusation could have justified his fury, because it is true; for some reason I never give Larry around-the-world. It's just one of those things. But I never kiss him, either, because his mouth doesn't turn me on. It is too thin and unsensuous.

But, as with all my personal lovers, I taught him how to make love properly and how to please a woman. However, I happen to like variety when I'm horny, and while I think I have made him understand this, it is impossible to make him accept it. Occasionally it drove him to fits of jealous anger. I was sure one of us would kill the other one day.

This almost happened in Puerto Rico one Christmas when Larry took me there for a week to rest and relax. We stayed at the El Conquistador, which is such a luxurious establishment that only very affluent older people and their young kids are there. A funicular train runs from the beach and pool up to the hotel. As far as action for me, there was nothing around except one beautiful-looking seventeen-year-old boy, tall as a sapling, with dark velvet eyes, sensuous, dramatic face, and that Continental-looking complexion that matched exactly with his longish golden-brown hair.

He was so gorgeous that I would think about him when Larry was making love to me.

But the closest we could get in the first couple of days was flirting across the casino tables under Larry's hawklike gaze, or splashing each other in the pool during the day.

On the third night, when I saw him appear immaculately dressed in a black velvet suit and black tie, I decided to do something about my passion for the kid. I engineered an argument with Larry at the tables. "Listen, you are losing too much money on the tables, so if you want to keep gambling, count me out. I'm going for a walk," I said, and left in a huff and rode the funicular down to the swimming pool, where I had already arranged to meet the kid.

When I arrived, I found he had his young brother with him, and he explained that his parents would not let one of them out without the other as chaperon.

Well, the two innocents lit up joints and started smoking them as we sat around the pool talking and kidding around. I was wearing a slinky décolleté dress, and the mosquitoes started biting my arms, so the kid gallantly suggested I go up to his room and protect myself. He was staying in his family's huge suite, so he had to smuggle me inside by checking first to see if they were asleep, then leading me on tiptoe to his room, where he bolted the door behind us.

The whole scene of seducing this beautiful young boy while his mommy and daddy slept unaware in the next room was very exciting.

As I started to undress, the kid wrapped his arms around me and engaged me in the most exotic kiss as he skillfully started from my shoulders.

When I was as bare as the day I was born, the kid lowered me onto the bed like priceless porcelain and took off his own clothes, revealing that beautiful chest on which the hairs were not completely grown. I had a tantalizing glimpse of his young, strong penis before he snapped out the light and joined me.

As in my early days in Puerto Rico when I taught all the young boys the art of love, I was prepared to show my present lover the way. But before I could assume a lead, he started caressing and kissing me in a way that would make Don Juan look like an amateur, and he ate pussy perfectly.

Half an hour later, after making love passionately, we lay relaxing, and my curiosity about the sexual skills of this baby got the better of me.

"Tell me, how come you know so much about making a woman happy at your age?" I asked curiously.

"My father is actually responsible for it in an indirect way," he told me. "You see, he came to visit me on the West Coast, where I am studying cinematography, and while there introduced me to his mistress.

"During the course of an evening he became involved in a business discussion with an associate, and his mistress and I were left to ourselves and soon became interested in each other.

"When my father returned east, warning me never to let my mother know about his girlfriend, she and I started seeing each other."

Although I had been careful to conceal my profession from the kid, he told me his father's mistress, whom he now secretly lived with, was a "business" girl and ten years older than himself.

As we talked lazily, I happened to look at my watch and discovered with horror that it was 4:00 A.M.—four hours since I had flounced out of the casino for a short walk.

"My God, I've got to get out of here!" I told my boy lover. "I've got a boyfriend waiting upstairs."

As I threw on my clothes the kid jumped into a pair of jeans, and, as any well-mannered man would do, insisted on escorting me home.

After waiting for the funicular for what seemed like an eternity, we rode up; we were to be confronted by the moon-washed outline of a very irate Larry standing on our balcony, which looked directly into each train car as it passed by.

There was no way he wouldn't spot us, and no way he wouldn't guess what we had been up to, since the kid was wearing a dinner suit when last seen, and suddenly he was in jeans.

We jumped off the funicular as it came to a halt, and hurried up to my floor. As we rounded the corridor corner, my bedroom door opened, and out into the hall came all my belongings—clothes, mirrors, brushes, combs, and luggage—onto the floor. I wouldn't be surprised if next came Larry with a knife in his hand, so I told the kid to vanish. "El splitto, go, don't hang around!" But Larry didn't appear in the hall. Instead the bedroom door slammed, and I could hear him yelling at the boy as he boarded the funicular. "You bastard, you had the nerve to fuck my wife. I'm going to tell your mother and father about this!" he screamed from the balcony at the top of his voice.

Lights of rudely awakened guests started peppering the front facade of the hotel, while meantime I was desperately trying to turn my key in the lock to get inside and shut Larry up. But he had jammed the keyhole with something.

As I poked and prodded, a well-dressed guest coming home late from the casino appeared in the hall.

"I'm sorry to trouble you, sir," I said, "but my lock seems to have stuck. I wonder, could you help me?"

The poor man looked a little tired, but he did his best to oblige. As he was bending down squinting into the stubborn lock, the door flew open to reveal a furious-faced Larry.

"You're trying to fuck my wife, too!" he accused the poor passerby. "I'll fix you all."

Suddenly, doors were opening, people stepped out into the hall, and it was excruciatingly embarrassing. I had to stop his paranoia at once, so I gave him a terrific shove back into the room, jumped inside, and slammed the door. Then the battle was on. We went for each other hammer and tongs, and I, being the stronger of the two, knocked Larry down onto the floor, grabbed his thick silver hair, and started pounding his head on the marble floor. One, two, three times I whammed it, until I realized that the next strike could kill him.

I saw a sudden fear of death in his eyes and only then did I realize what a crime of passion exactly meant. People who are so enraged and strong don't know when to stop beating each other up.

I let him up on the promise he would calm down and not mention the incident again. I spent the rest of the night trying to placate him, and the next morning we decided to move out of the hotel, taking the 7:00 A.M. helicopter down to the El San Juan.

Larry eventually got over the incident and forgave me. When I am horny I have to find a victim; besides, those episodes are like ships that pass in the night. It's the ships that dock for a while that really drive him mad. I occasionally have an affair with a man I might meet on the job that could go on for weeks or months.

Last winter I fell in love with a thirty-three-year-old banker named Skip, who looked like Sean Connery in his younger years. Larry knew about it, but accepted the situation as long as the man paid me. If there was a check from him in the morning when Larry came by, he would feel reassured, but if it was missing he would be angry. Which is hypocritical, in a way, because I could still love my banker whether he paid me or not. Although sometimes I love to mix emotions with physical pleasure and business, and Skip used to pay a considerable sum to spend the night with me. He was very handsome with a fantastic body, and a great sense of humor.

Skip used to come by around 9:00 P.M., mingle with the group of people in the living room, tease the girls, and drive them out of their mind—since he knew he was a good-looking flirt, being very conceited indeed. At times he would parade around the house in one of Larry's silk robes, and while chatting on the couch, he would reveal certain parts of his body by letting it drop open halfway "accidentally." All my girls liked him, and if it wasn't for my house rule, the code of ethics—"Don't touch Madam Xaviera's lover"—they sure as hell would have liked to make a pass at him "for free."

While being with Skip, I didn't care for anyone else, and it was a divine feeling to really love someone again. During peak hours he would jokingly help me out by serving drinks to my thirsty customers, and walk around with a white towel on his sleeve as if he really were the butler. In between we would make love and have long, sentimental conversations.

Skip's favorite thirst quencher was beer. I can't remember how many dozens of cans of beer I got him during those months we saw each other. He would even send my maid out to get it, and give her a generous tip afterward.

However, my James Bond was even more jealous than Larry. If Skip was in the house, I was not even allowed to close the bedroom door and discuss, in private, finances with my customers, since he thought I would make it with that man. Nor could I "chip in" on a swing or a threesome without Skip immediately threatening to walk out on me. Granted that I might have lost some income by giving up these extra activities, but Skip's overall generosity, his fine body and mind—not to speak of the many red roses he sent—gave me quite some happiness for several months. Finally a combination of family problems and business pressures reduced our relationship to one of friendship, but we remain good friends, and there is still a warm and tender feeling for each other.

As Skip was sent sailing off, another ship docked, tied up, and looked as though it was here to stay. A Greek boy, Takis, about twenty-nine, came to see me about two girls he wanted me to meet. They were from Montreal, he said, and wanted to become my roommates. The doorbell rang, and here was this gorgeous young man built like an Adonis, dark hair, and green eyes exactly the same color as mine, except that he has got long black eyelashes. He has a baby smile on his sensuous, dramatic face. Only his nose is a bit small, in my opinion, definitely non-Greek.

Takis and I caught fire from that very first moment we met. We made love almost immediately after his appearance, and he then more or less moved into my life and my penthouse apartment. The ship had docked. His tongue was warm and fast, and, I must confess, there has been no feeling nicer than having this Greek boy giving me head. He also knew exactly where to touch my body, blow kisses on my neck, and make love to me. Our rhythm was that of the ever-moving waves of the ocean. Come and go, up and down, back and forth. That's how his lovemaking affected me.

Takis, a very emotional and sensitive person, as it turned out, became one of the sweetest things in my life. He was good, kind, never impolite or rude. He was lazy in a way, since he loved to sleep late in the day, but so did my roommates, the two Canadians he had meanwhile introduced to me. They also had moved in with me, and all of a sudden the house was full of laughter and happy young people. Takis, to my knowledge, had never slept with either of the two Canadians. He had told me that in Montreal he used to be the boyfriend of a rather well-known Madam Carmine. So, in other words, he was used to the late hours, the many different men who came to patronize the house of Carmine. She had been in this business about ten years and managed to save a good deal of money, with which she was said to be rather generous.

Being Greek, Takis had one of the famous Greek weaknesses, and that was gambling. He would not, like most men might do, cheat on his girlfriend, but the few nights that he did come home in the early-morning hours he always confessed to me that he had gone to some after-hours gambling joint, where prefer-ably his favorite Armenian game of *barbout*, a game similar to crap shooting, was played. Takis was constantly broke. I used to support him, not in great sums like Carmine allegedly did, but with a $10 or $20 bill here and there. One night when he left, all he had in his pocket was $12, but when he came home at ten the next day, he was exhausted but very satisfied—he showed me proudly how he had won with his small sum the big sum of $2,000.

However, the money seemed somehow to burn the proverbial hole in his pocket, and like a masochist he had to go back to the tables and lose it all. Since it was not actually money from my savings or anything like that, I could never really get mad at him. Of course, I wished he would save his winnings or get a steady job, but lazy as he was at that time, he preferred to be the boyfriend, almost gigololike, of Madam Xaviera. Not that he ever purposely took advantage of me—that I can guarantee. It was always my own idea when I decided to be generous with him. And he never *asked* for a thing. Some days I would take him downtown and buy him some new shirts or some Jockey underpants or a nice woolen sweater that revealed his sexy body even more. All this while, we really were tremendously turned on by each other, and used to make love night after night till sunup.

It didn't take Larry long to realize that my Greek boy who acted as bartender and played gin rummy with the customers was actually living in the apartment.

"Have you fucked Xaviera, Takis?" Larry asked bluntly on more than one occasion.

"Oh, no, of course not," Takis would answer. "We are friends. I am happy to get the work and a place to sleep."

I always denied that I made love to Takis, but Larry, of course, knew me too well to believe it, and finally, stupidly, I admitted that Takis and I did it. I am too honest to be able to lie.

When Larry heard this, he virtually threw Takis and me out of my own house, stating that since the apartment lease was in his name, I had no right to put another man in the house.

That morning, like a beaten-up dog, my Greek packed his one big suitcase and I checked him into a little hotel not too far away from where I lived. I paid the bill for the coming week, and at night he would sneak back into my house, when he knew that the coast was clear and that no jealous maniac, namely Larry, was there anymore.

This was an impossible situation, and it was ridiculous to pay a hotel on the side, while he, as a matter of fact, was still spending every night except the weekends—then Larry was there—with me. After a week I said to Takis, "This is crazy. Let's stop throwing money away on the hotel. We'll face reality and tell Larry he can't stop us from being together anymore."

I decided to tell Larry about our deep feelings for each other. Amazingly, Larry took the news very bravely, almost fatherlike, although it was hard for him to accept the three-way situation. Once again he was being cheated with his eyes wide open. His ego was crushed, and, what's more, he liked Takis, who is truly an amiable person. Still, Larry couldn't really blame me for being in love with this gorgeous boy so much younger than he, and finally agreed to accept the situation so long as I didn't treat him badly or embarrass him in front of other people.

The high—or low—point of this uneasy triangle came when we spent a summer weekend at the beach home of friends in Westhampton, Long Island. Larry and I had a bedroom together, with an adjoining bathroom, and beyond the bathroom was the bedroom given to Takis.

The first night, as soon as I thought Larry was asleep, I sneaked into the bathroom, locked the door to Larry's and my room, and went into Takis's room. But Larry was *not* asleep and was listening at the bathroom door. Takis and I were so horny, I first gave him a blow job, and as I later found out, Larry heard me washing my mouth out afterward. Then he even heard when I put my diaphragm in and went back to Takis for my straight lovemaking. When I finally returned to the room I shared with

Larry, he was furious. We had a big fight, and he threatened to walk out. While I didn't want to lose Larry, I could understand that the weekend was going to be a depressing experience for him if I was horny for Takis all the time. We went to bed, still together, but still upset. Whatever I do, it is not in my mind ever consciously to hurt Larry.

The next day Takis, in a very suave and civilized manner, asked why we couldn't lead a three-way relationship—in other words, why *can't* two men love one woman at the same time? Often a man has an affair with two girls, he reasoned. Why not vice versa? However, even for me, working out this arrangement was a very weird experience. Larry gave in to it because there was no way out. He knew I would choose Takis if I were forced to pick between them, and he did not want to lose me completely, I guess.

So on Sunday morning we decided to make our strange little *ménage à trois* start to work. The weather at the beach wasn't too good that day, and not many people were out. We walked down to a secluded part of the beach, where nobody was in sight, the sun was behind a heavy cloud cover, and we put a towel down on the sand.

I lay in the middle of the big beach towel, and Larry rolled my bikini down a bit and began to play with my clitoris. My head was resting on Takis's lap, and I could feel his powerful hard-on against my shoulder. He was caressing my breasts and kissing my mouth. I never kiss Larry, as I have mentioned, but Takis has the most sensuous mouth, and a beautiful way of kissing me. Soon I was having a delicious climax, wriggling like crazy all over the two of them, although at the same time I was also conscious that I was being selfish, since the two men had not been able to enjoy the same pleasure all the way.

After this beautiful one-way sex ritual with my two lovers, I noticed what was going on around me. Several men had pulled their beach chairs closer to us and were looking our way through their sunglasses. It was time to leave. People were getting too curious. We decided to drive back to the city late that afternoon, and I thought it would be nice to give both of them a blow job on the way back. But they were both too embarrassed to expose themselves in front of each other, so I ended up putting my head on Larry's lap while he drove, and my toes teased Takis's prick. Back in New York we all had dinner together, and then Larry had to go home to visit his kids. By then Larry had realized I was in love with Takis, my steady paramour now.

"Good night, Takis. Have a nice evening," Larry ground out between his teeth when we parted. He gave me a bitter smile.

It was all very complicated, because I really hated to hurt Larry in any way. After all, we had been together for so long. So I instructed both my lovers that I want no more scenes.

And so we settled down to a routine. I would make love to Larry about once a week, but always with the door tightly closed or when Takis was sound asleep. But, ironically, it was the turn of Takis to become jealous when I would swing, which I did just for kicks. When he learned of one of my escapades, he was furious and would not make love to me for several days.

I recalled how one of my earliest boyfriends in Holland would declare "I give you my sperm, I give you my soul" whenever we made love. But he told me that he fucked other girls, but to them he gave only his sperm, so that he was never guilty of actually cheating on me. I endeavored to expound this philosophy to Larry and Takis—and to many subsequent lovers. For me, loving is a complete giving and taking of soul, mind, and body. Anything less is just the meeting of two ships that pass in the night.

Seventeen

Abe the Bugger

Abe the Bugger was the cause of my less-active days as a New York madam.

Abe's real identity will be apparent to anyone who read the papers in 1971 or watched the television reports on police corruption in New York and my own part in the controversial hearings of the Knapp Commission appointed by Mayor John Lindsay to study corruption in New York City's government and police department.

Abe is one of those electronic geniuses who can bug anything: apartments, phones, offices, or cars. He was introduced to me by my coauthor, Robin Moore, who wanted to have Abe install a tape-recorder system in my bedroom in order to get authenticity for this book.

Abe the Bugger is not an easy person to describe in words. He must be seen to be believed. Think of 190 pounds of fat held in a five-foot-six body. Cover this with a baby-pink wrapping; add two thick, ever moist lips, and dot with powder-blue eyes—each forever magnified by a couple of Coca-Cola bottle bottoms for glasses—all sitting under three strands of hair assigned the impossible task of covering something that only a loving mother could call a head. Then you might have a feeling for Abe the Bugger.

Perhaps because he thinks his eighteen-month jail sentence a few years ago was unjustified, Abe's seeming ambition in life is to turn up evidence against crooked political figures and judges. He was constantly assuring me that today he leads a perfectly straight life, saving pennies and living on what he makes as an investigator. Indeed, he reminded me of nothing more than a bad penny, always turning up at the wrong moment.

But of course once Abe was in, he really was in. First, he wired most of my telephones and connected them to a huge tape recorder hidden in my closet. At this moment I had second thoughts. "But I thought that we were going to have one of those small tape recorders that I simply turn on and off!" I told him.

"No, no, no, Robin wants all the sound," Abe insisted.

Abe the Bugger was Robin's man. How could I, madam though I may be, ever confuse artistry with art?

"How about the switch?" I pursued. "Listen, I want to be able to turn this thing off."

"Okay," he said. "Here is the switch. Press it here and it goes on, and press it there and off it goes. So you see, now you can record any conversation you want, and if you don't want to record it, you don't even have to put it on," he replied with a cherubic smile.

Like Pandora's box, Abe, once turned on, was evil energy unleashed. "Your phones . . ."

"What about my phones?" I asked.

"They could be bugged."

"Oh?"

"I will check them out." And check them out he did. I have never seen such activity. Electronic gadgets with all sorts of flicking lights and purring noises.

"Aha, it *is* bugged. You got a bug here."

"Where?"

"Don't worry, don't worry, I know."

"How? How do you know?"

"The . . . [a spew forth of words I knew to be English but that sounded more like Einstein going mad] . . . and when it registers on this meter, I know there is a bug."

"Okay. There is a bug." I mean, who the hell could argue, anyway?

"Aha [*click, click, push, pull, click click*] . . . and this one has a pen register."

"How the hell? Never mind . . . What the hell is a pen register?"

He told me it records all the numbers dialed. I wanted to know what I should do. He quickly explained; there was that smile again. I was to do nothing, he would do it all. He opened up another black box with meters and lights, and after half an hour's work he sighed in satisfaction. "No more bug. I have just burned it off. It will take them ten days to get a court order to put a new one on. As for the pen-register phone, just use it for incoming calls or to call out for shopping or food deliveries or general chitchat talk with friends."

The tape recorder was fun. I spent the next few days taping some of the phone calls and interviewing some friends and johns. Of course, I would ask them for their permission first and keep their identity unknown.

Once again, Abe came to visit. Not satisfied with having a bug in the bedroom, he wanted to bug the sounds of the living room as well.

"No good," I said. I thought that this was carrying reality too far, since I would certainly lose control in a big group of people. It was not till very much later I learned that Abe had put a tiny but powerful radio transmitter in the back of the night table next to my bed, and every sound in my bedroom could be picked up and broadcast to another tape recorder in an office a block from my apartment building, whether I pressed the switch or not.

Abe, it seems, had a sideline: selling information to law-enforcement agencies and others. I found out about the hidden bug and Abe's sideline only when Knapp Commission investigators called me as a witness many months later. They had in their possession tapes made in my apartment without my knowledge or consent. So our Abe the Bugger was a busy bug indeed. Carried away with his hidden electronic gadgets, he went even further.

About two months after Abe made his first appearance at my place, he showed up on a periodic visit to check my phones for "taps." On this visit he burned off "a new one" for a quick $250 and, unbeknown to me, left behind another gadget.

Approximately two weeks later, Larry was pouring liquor from half-gallon bottles into smaller bottles and straightening up my place when he suddenly called me into the bedroom. He told me to stand on a chair and look at the back of the round golden mirror hanging above my bed. There in the middle of the back of the mirror was a little black metal box.

Abe, you son of a bitch, what the hell does this mean? I thought to myself. Larry gave a whistle and pulled the box off the mirror. We then put it away in my closet. Abe would have some explaining to do.

"It's nothing," he said the following day. That same smile again. "Just a booster for the tape recorder." It was not until months later that Robin told me I had been on television.

It turned out that the box was a television camera which worked something like radar. A laser beam directed at the camera in my apartment from a nearby office activated the black box and relayed pictures to the sophisticated receiving equipment in Abe's office. Good old businesslike Abe had not only been listening to what went on in my apartment, he was watching as well. What he did was play with the dials of the big TV instrument in his office until he brought in the picture from my bedroom, and then sat down to watch, that liver-lipped little voyeur.

But Abe wasn't as smart as he thought he was. After all his work, he watched me in action for a total of only forty-five minutes. The picture actually got picked up and appeared on one of New York's commercial UHF channels, a Spanish-language station, I believe. And these viewers, I gather, got to watch quite an orgy for forty-five minutes.

When the F.B.I. was called in to investigate, the agents immediately assumed that only one person was capable of so sophisticated an electronic stunt. They called Abe in and threatened him with everything in the book if he did such a thing again, and I guess they scared him pretty badly.

To say the least, Abe is well known to the F.B.I. and the various crime commissions operating in New York, and has sold information to them. Soon after he met me he suggested that I make payoffs to stay in business. Truthfully, it was difficult for me to go for more than four or five months without getting busted under normal circumstances, and he claimed that payoffs would ease this situation.

Abe admitted to me that he was doing work for two crime

commissions investigating corruption. He also told me that anything I did to help this work was strictly a favor, and I could expect help in return.

Abe did indeed introduce me to State Senator John H. Hughes and his legal counsel, Edward McLaughlin. Senator Hughes heads a committee in Albany—the weighty full title of which is the New York State Joint Legislative Committee on Crime, Its Causes, Control, and Effect on Society—and he and his counsel offered me help with my immigration case in return for my future cooperation. I am always worried about being deported—with good reason, I'm afraid—and I believed that Abe really could speak on Senator Hughes's behalf.

However, I never completely trusted the bugger. Even though he pretended to be such a good friend of the house, why then the "friendly" fees of $200 or $300? For burning off the supposedly existing wiretaps on my phones? Where was the *prix d'amis*?

One day I went to meet a friend at a lawyer's office before lunchtime. I knew the lawyer, Ed Carmino, from years before. I'd never really cared for Carmino—he was too slick and dealt with too many creepy individuals, and I would definitely regard him as a "shyster" lawyer. I chatted with Carmino a few minutes before my friend took me out for lunch, and I happened to mention my problem of having been arrested several times in the past months. Carmino immediately said he would introduce me that night to someone who might be of help to me.

Sure enough, late that afternoon a visitor was announced by my doorman as a friend of Mr. Carmino. When I opened the door I found a tall, thin, black-haired man who perhaps was in his early forties. Smiling, he identified himself, and since he was both pleasant and well dressed, I led him in. Bill Phillips, as he had introduced himself, then further identified himself as a plainclothes detective who felt he should help me, since I was a friend of Ed Carmino. He showed me his badge and I.D. card, and I wrote down the numbers.

We then discussed the fact that the "heat" was on. Mayor Lindsay's crackdown on prostitution had not only curtailed street prostitution but also private call girls and the houses run by various madams. The busts had been frequent, and in March 1971, I was thrown into jail together with one of my German girls and an innocent roommate. The case was still pending, and it looked rather gloomy, since my biggest fear was a conviction, even if it was only for loitering for "the purpose of prostitution." Anything regarded as moral turpitude could prevent my getting the all-important U.S. resident's green card that I had been awaiting for so long. Of course, I mentioned this to Bill, and he asked me who the arresting officer had been in my case. I told him, and we left it at that. Bill then took me for a drink at P. J. Clarke's, my favorite hangout, just around the corner from where I was then living. At P. J.'s Bill seemed to know everyone, and people kept coming over to our table, kidding around and buying us drinks. Mine were soft drinks, as usual, but Bill had several free belts. Bill and I finally made a date to meet with my boyfriend the next day at my house to discuss where to go next to solve my problem.

That evening both Larry and Abe were at the apartment, and I mentioned the meeting with Bill. Abe immediately became very interested and said that since he was in a position to check out cops better than Larry and me, we should let *him* pose as my boyfriend, meet Bill, and act as my intermediary in whatever proposal Bill might make. He, meanwhile, jotted down the numbers I had copied from Bill's badge and identification card, and left to check those out.

So, two days later when Bill came up to the apartment, Abe was there. Ugh! I hated even to introduce Abe as my boyfriend, since the thought of having him as a boyfriend almost made me puke. However, Abe and Bill seemed to get along well, and before I even could open my mouth, they'd made a deal for monthly payoffs of $1,100 to the police for protection.

When I complained about the high monthly figure, Abe told me I'd better cooperate, since I needed the protection, or else I would get deported. So I kept quiet, and, to cement the deal, I treated Bill to one of my girls.

The next day Bill introduced three police officers from the precinct to Abe at P. J.'s, which had now become our regular meeting place. Bill was one of the smartest and biggest bagmen in New York, Abe told me later. Most of the big payoffs went through him. Abe added that Bill probably put half the money he collected in his own pocket. Moreover, according to Abe, Bill owned three airplanes and an expensive house.

Larry and I decided to convince ourselves we had confidence in this new arrangement. Actually, we had no alternative but to cooperate, and Abe did seem reliable as long as I handed over the $1,100 each month. Things went along well for about three months with Abe and Bill being thick as thieves—which of course they indeed were.

Meanwhile, another "deal" was made. This had to do with my previous arrest. After discussions back and forth with Abe and the arresting police officer, Bill fixed a price of $3,500 to get me off the hook completely. Originally the arresting officer had suggested wryly that the "golden goose" ought to pay $10,000 to get her case dismissed, but as that figure was rather outrageous, they settled for $3,500. Again, there was really nothing I could do about it other than get up the money. Later on I found out that only $1,500 was being paid to the arresting officer. What happened to the rest of the money, only Abe and Bill know!

After all this was taken care of, my case still had not been thrown out completely, since my lawyer, properly straitlaced, refused to cooperate in a bribe case and pleaded me guilty of a misdemeanor: loitering. I got off with a $100 fine, but it wasn't the money that hurt, it was the police card in my name.

One day Abe came to Larry and asked for a large favor. The favor—and the word is used loosely—involved a situation in which Larry had got himself involved in connection with an allegedly stolen insurance check involving a considerable sum. Abe said he'd looked into the case and had spoken to the assistant district attorney handling the case. And Larry would have a great opportunity to do a tremendous amount of good for the crime committee, Abe told him, if he cooperated in the following manner: Larry's case was to be handled by a very prominent New York judge whom the committee was then investigating. The judge was very close to a certain lawyer, who was none other than Ed Carmino. Abe wanted Larry to please go along with the farce of employing Ed Carmino as his attorney and having him try to fix the case via a payoff.

Although Larry had his own attorney and was quite prepared to go to court, he decided to go along with the game. Among other things, he was promised by Abe that he'd get the "payoff" money back, since it was being used to gain an indictment of the judge.

The next few days, Bill and Abe put their heads together with the lawyer, Carmino, to discuss the "fixing" of Larry's case. Abe came back and told me that he would need $10,000 to "take care" of my boyfriend's case. I told him that I did not have that kind of money, since I had just been arrested and had a steep lawyer's bill myself. Also, I'd just laid out a lot of money in my own case.

Besides all this, my business was rather slow at that time, what with my publicized arrest and the summer months coming up, when most people leave town. And why should I let Abe and Bill bleed me to death anyway? To cooperate with a crime committee—well, fine! But to what extent? How could I trust this crazy situation?

Abe then became very "moral" and insinuated that my money was ill-gotten anyway. "Easy come, easy go." So why shouldn't I lend Larry, who had been my steady boyfriend for the past year, the $10,000 to make the payoff to the bagman? "You don't want your boyfriend to get in trouble, do you?" he asked sarcastically. In other words, Abe put the knife to my throat, threatening me again with deportation and arrest. Still, $10,000 to me was not exactly peanuts, although my monthly $1,100 was not petty cash either.

Being very persuasive, Abe swore that I would get all the money back later, although the crime commission did not have sufficient funds available just then. Finally it was agreed that Larry and I would split the $10,000 and each put $5,000 up. Larry spent a lot of time on taking down the serial numbers from the $100 bills that we gave Abe, who assured us that he would be able to trace our money both by the serial numbers and additional unseen markings that he would put on himself.

Larry went with Abe to Carmino's office, where discussions took place as to how to pay off the judge.

Two weeks later Bill came dashing up to my apartment. He was yelling-screaming mad about "that bastard Abe." He ranted: "I always did wonder about him and his neat suits and ties, carrying his attaché case in the middle of this hot summer weather."

What happened was that after every payment Abe made for me at P. J. Clarke's, he would lead Bill into talking about who the payoffs were going to and who on the police force was taking bribes. When Abe went to meet Carmino with Bill, as usual he was immaculately dressed, with his suit buttoned, and carrying, as ever, his briefcase.

Bill had noticed how Abe nonchalantly waved his briefcase around when he was talking in the lawyer's office. He became suspicious when Abe made Ed Carmino repeat the name of the prominent judge several times. Bill had suddenly grabbed Abe from behind, pulled his coat off, and found the man was completely wired. Everything that was said had gone into the little microphone Abe wore. I now recalled that Abe had confessed to me once that his little black attaché case was equipped with cameras, and the lens shutter worked by moving the handle up and down. Without even opening the case, he could shoot as many pictures as he wanted.

According to Bill's story, Carmino was so outraged that he pulled a gun from his drawer and threatened Abe with it. Just then two men came bursting into the office. They identified themselves as agents from the Knapp Commission. Obviously the two agents came just in time to prevent harm to anyone, and now came the moment of revelation. All this time Abe had not been representing Senator Hughes's Committee on Crime in Albany, but rather the Knapp Commission. Even though I lost several thousand dollars, I couldn't help laughing at myself for having been actually financing Mayor Lindsay's crime commission in one of its biggest investigations.

Meanwhile, Bill accused me of knowing all about Abe's working with the Knapp Commission, and I had to keep denying it in the worst way, since I really had not been aware of it. So, willingly or unwillingly, I suppose I have been of quite some help to the Knapp Commission.

As far as I myself am concerned, I was highly surprised to read that Abe had accused me of having blackmailed, bribed, and extorted money from my customers, and even of being involved with drugs. This is all untrue, and there was a possibility of Abe himself being indicted for his activities. In the meantime, heavy investigations continued, and I was called in daily to the New York district attorney's office for what information I could provide.

Meanwhile, Abe, whose house was raided by the New York district attorney, was left helpless without his gadgets and tape recordings, his decoder and descrambler, his burning-off device, and the other tools of his nefarious trade. At the same time, my girls were being harassed with obscene telephone calls, and I know Abe photostated my address books. It may be their imaginations, but some of my girls said they recognized his voice from hearing him on a television interview recently.

30 Years Later

9 would like to feel that all those payoffs, legal fees, and fines were worthwhile because the world after *The Happy Hooker* was that much freer and less prudish.

But is that how things really seem today? On the plus side, women involved in the sex industry can claim the same respect as any other workers. They are no longer expected to feel shame for being paid for providing an essential service. Indeed, they actively organize to defend their rights as effectively as any labor union or political pressure group, and organizations like the International Sex Worker Foundation for Art, Culture and Education (ISWFACE) are helping to promote art, culture, and books by and about sex workers. And with the growing number of financially independent women who are able to choose their own lifestyles, women can openly buy sexual services as well as sell them, allowing male prostitutes to share the enhanced status achieved by their sister workers, jettisoning the shopworn image of the gigolo. That's my idea of equality!

This recognition was summed up eloquently by one acknowledged authority in sexual counseling, Dr. Patti Britton:

> Sex workers have been an astute source of referral to me for clients seeking sexual counseling or therapy. . . . Most of the sex workers with whom I've consulted showed an impressive range of personal characteristics, such as being empowered about their own business capacity; comfortable with their bodies, the man's body, and their own sexuality; being clear about setting goals and boundaries with clients; being caring and compassionate, especially about the men who suffered from lack of social skills or persistent sexual problems; being bright and articulate; being open to treatment options, especially in working with my male clients who suffered from persistent challenges with erectile difficulties (pre-Viagra) and ejaculatory control issues (also pre-medications).
>
> My personal dream for the world is that the hatred and misunderstanding of professional sex workers will disappear. I advocate the legalization of prostitution. I support the elevation of the status of sex workers, many of whom offer the sole place in the life of a man for touch, love and compassion. I hope that the world will eventually open itself to support the flourishing of sexual pleasure in all of its dimensions—whether with a loving, lifelong, committed partner, or with a paid hour of touching in the healing presence of a sex worker. To me sex workers include strippers, phone sex workers, Internet performers, XXX actors, sexual surrogates, prostitutes, sexual escorts, dominatrixes, and all others who perform the delicate and demanding tasks of providing service to others with their bodies, their minds, and often their hearts. I salute them all.

It so happens that Dr. Britton is my cousin: it's good to have such unanimity within the family! Yet there are still battles to be won. As one highly trained and sensitive social worker wrote me, "When I do counseling I hear the same themes of alienation, which I believe is more of a problem here in America because we work illegally, and our culture tends to stigmatize sexuality more than Europe does."

Nevertheless, I find today that sex is well and truly out of the closet. There is a thriving pornography industry, to such an extent that words or pictures once considered so naughty that the zealots of upright, uptight America howled for them to be banned are now commonplace and no longer shocking. In reaction, of course, publishers produce more and more explicit, in-your-face material—but often eroticism is replaced by mindless violence. I don't go for that sort of sensationalism. It seems like the new slogan is "Make war, not love!" Where has all the humor gone?

Inevitably, the demented screams of the religious right have also taken on the same offensively violent tone. Television preachers bang the Bible with one hand while raking in the dollars with the other. And they can pull all the political strings: the holier-than-thou evangelicals have even captured the White House! *Maxim, Gear, Stuff*, and *FHM* are fun magazines that show sexy pictures of models and film and television stars, yet so insidious is the power of the puritan backlash that they refuse to show a female nipple lest they be dropped from major retail chain stores across the country. I guess sex in America these days is the same old story: confusion, anxiety, titillation, experimentation, and danger, danger everywhere. The American reactionary backlash against sexuality in our new century focuses on danger: AIDS, date rape, teenage pregnancy, abortion, sexual harassment, child molestation, and pornography. Fifteen years ago, in an earlier reissue of this book, I asked, "Can it be that the first edition of *The Happy Hooker* marked the end of a dark age, only for this edition to be greeted by a return to the hypocrisy and persecution that we thought had been vanquished? Or will American common sense and goodwill prevail?" Maybe the jury is still out.

Then, of course, came September 11th, and Americans woke up to the fact that during wartime each moment might be their last—and so might each fuck. The business of sex had a new relevance. Here is one account that was sent to me:

Since the events of September 11th, I have found an interesting anomaly in the daily operations of my two legal brothels, the Moonlite Bunnyranch and Miss Kitty's Pussycat Lounge. Though business has remained steady, there have been an exceptionally large number of first-time customers visiting both brothels. The girls have confided in me that for many of these gentlemen this is indeed their first visit to a brothel—and what's compelled them is that [the need for] intimate physical contact has become more urgent since the tragedy in New York City.

These clients seem to feel that the bar of morality has been raised to a higher level—that how a woman chooses to make an honest living is her business, and how a fellow spends his money is an equally personal decision. Some guys who have been saving for trips or cars or other material items are cashing in for the instant gratification of sexual satisfaction and the company of a warm body. Others have decided that rather than playing the odds of the singles pick-up scene—engaging in mundane small talk designed to get into some gal's pants—they'll simply take the direct route: it's a more real and honest relationship that comes with no baggage, breakups, or pregnancies.

The girls tell me that many of these men are going for fantasies they've long harbored but never realized, deciding it may be unwise to put off these cravings any longer but unwilling to risk the rejection or rebuff of a girlfriend or wife. Therefore, they're reaching out to professionals who will not pass judgment on their particular peccadilloes.

Quite frankly, I think the girls are getting into it as well. The idea, though overly dramatic, that each fuck might be the last, that the personal stake is somehow higher than normal, makes for a very good vibe, and an extremely hot level of sex.

It's ironic that it takes a tragedy of such epic proportions to sort of shuffle the deck of decency and self-righteousness, and allow people to focus on common evils rather than pedestrian hang-ups. The value of flesh on flesh, of lips pressing, of two consenting adults reaching orgasmic oblivion, is getting its richly deserved place on the mantle of human experience.

I know from my own childhood experience of war that the shock of atrocities wears off, that people become accustomed to living in fear, so I wonder whether life at the Bunnyranch and Miss Kitty's will gradually slip back to a more casual brand of peacetime service. Without wanting to prolong the sense of crisis, though, I can't help feeling that if that sense of urgency disappears, something precious will have been lost.

However, the movement for openness and honesty has certainly spread to many other countries: the message of this book, in the current jargon, has gone global. To take just one example, one lifestyle dominatrix and writer living and working in Sydney, Australia, wrote to tell me that before 1979, when prostitution was decriminalized, street prostitutes were arrested every week and all the sex establishments paid the police $150 a week to stay open. So corrupt was the system that even then at least one staff member would be arrested each week to keep the arrest rates high. Today Sydney's sex industry is one of the safest in the world, with the lowest rates of HIV and STD infection of any Western country, including Holland. And while I was on a visit to Scotland, I heard an interview on the BBC's quality news channel with the leader of Britain's Collective of Prostitutes, who was treated with complete seriousness and respect.

And in what surely must be the ultimate triumph, the world's oldest profession has won limited approval from the European Union's highest court. The Court of Human Rights in Luxembourg has ruled that a group of Eastern European women has the right to work as prostitutes in the Netherlands. The case involved six Polish and Czech women working as window prostitutes in Amsterdam who'd been denied residence permits that would allow them to work on a self-employed basis, on the grounds that prostitution is not a regular job or profession. The court ruled that prostitutes could work in EU countries where selling sex is tolerated, as long as they have sufficient financial resources to carry out their activity and a reasonable chance of success. Prostitution, in their words, is "a service provided for remuneration." We knew that all along—after all, even judges were among my clients in the days (or rather, nights) when I provided that service "for remuneration." But now it's official.

In the United States, the Happy Hooker's homeland, an entire generation of Happy Hooker protegées has emerged, and the Hooker has become such an icon in her own right—quite separate from the real-life me—that she has appeared in the lives of fictional characters in books by other people. And, according to a newspaper report from Wellington, New Zealand, that was recently forwarded to me, "The United States remains the sexual superpower of the world, with Americans making love more often and with more partners than any other nationality, according to a survey by a leading condom manufacturer."

That seems to be a suitably upbeat note on which to put this revised edition of *The Happy Hooker* to bed—has that expression ever been used more appropriately?

—Xaviera Hollander, June 2002